The Garden of Being

Author

Denise Hammerberg (1961-2008) - "Dede" lived life with bravado and endless curiosity. She began writing after receiving a stage IV life alter-cancer diagnosis. After her memoir (The Garden of Being) was in print, she was recruited for speaking engagements related to the book's theme. She inspired many others with her courage and spirit of sharing. She chose the word "*Bloom*" as her byline and affirmation of life.

book available at www.amazon.com

email inquiries: darksey@charter.net

Published by Two Voices Publishing, LLC, Lapeer MI USA

Visit

The Garden of Being

book available at

www.amazon.com

BE

Email: darksey@yahoo.com

DENISE HAMMERBERG &
DOLLY ARKSEY

THE GARDEN OF BEING

2007

The Garden of Being

CONTENTS

ACKNOWLEDGEMENTS

Our sincere thanks and affection go to the following people for assisting with editing and providing generous quantities of inspiration on an "as needed" basis:

Cindy Arksey
Richard Arksey
Carolyn Jones
Dorcas McIntosh

A special thank you goes to our artist and illustrator, Michael Monville, who, like us, was sailing into unknown waters with this project. Michael contributed much more than drawings and art; he kept our spirits buoyed and tackled each image with the highest degree of sensitivity as to what each image conveyed about certain aspects of our story. Mike is a masterful artist and we are grateful for his generosity of time and talent to provide visual 'communication' along with the story.

Our appreciation to those people who shared hugs and words of encouragement throughout this 'journey' will be endless.

Dedicated To Life And Perpetual Gardens

INTRODUCTION

A book is like a garden carried in the pocket.
—Chinese Proverb

This is a story of a poignant and turbulent year in the lives of a daughter, who was found to have a serious form of breast cancer, and her mother that inspired both of them to think of life as living every day in a garden, The Garden of Being.

This story begins with the shocking and unwelcome news that cancer had made an unexpected call. The story is told through two voices. One is the voice of Denise (called Dede by her family), the daughter, now in her forties, who has been told by her doctor that she has stage IV cancer. The other voice is her mother, Dolly, now in her sixties. These two voices relate trauma and triumph over the course of almost one year. Dede, the indomitable "warrior", with her troops of dedicated family, friends, doctors and nurses, and "Momma" Dolly, who is taking the same garden path walk to be beside her daughter every step of the way. Each chapter gives a separate accounting of their thoughts and observations on shared or closely connected events along the way. The chapters are planted with an abundance of human drama—fear, dismay, tears, elation, joy, laughter (good medicine), and love (best medicine). It is a telling look inside the human heart.

Recollections are told in two voices and represented as follows: MD (Momma Dolly) and DD (Daughter Denise "Dede").

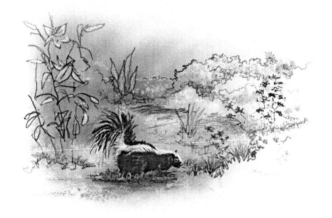

1

Unwelcome Visitor

MD:

News of an intruder into our lives came by a phone call from our daughter, Denise, in the month of June 2006. Her father and I were anticipating her call with high optimism and expecting good news. We were hopeful that results of her recent surgery to have an acorn-size lump from the left side of her neck removed would show the mass to be benign as had been the case with two earlier such occurrences. Over the past three years there had been a lump in her left breast and one in her lower back that had tested as non-cancerous. It was almost getting routine; perhaps it was a fibroid-prone affliction.

This time the message was heart-stopping. The lump tested positive. That was not the total message. The tests showed cancerous cells in the lymph nodes and evidence that this disease had originated in the breast and metastasized to other organs. Denise was telling us on the phone in her typical straightforward "tell it like it is" manner, but I could hear the breaking tone and quaver in her words. She told us she and Ken, our son-in-law, would be over shortly. This was definitely a time and moment that she needed to feel our love; and we needed to put our arms around her and let our energies and commitment flow through us to her and back again.

It seemed for a while that time stood still like in a bad dream and this was not real. Dede (our pet name for Denise) had been so careful about monitoring her health with yearly physicals and mammograms. It seemed absurd that this could happen so fast without a doctor or a test revealing the disease that had been speeding through her body so quickly under the surface, hiding like a thief beneath a bed under her ever present bright smiles, twinkling eyes and love of life. Her laugh is like no other. Like a mother hen who can find her own little chick in a gathering of hundreds, I could find her easily by hearing her laughter among a hundred other busy sounds.

An earlier emotional and frightening experience from 1973 came flooding over my brain as I set the phone down after the phone call. It was when Dede was twelve. After a physical exam done prior to a scheduled tonsillectomy (that was cancelled upon the news) it was discovered that she had a heart murmur/malfunction that would require surgery to correct. As a parent, your whole being feels like it's on meltdown and you can only throw yourself into the hands of nature's grace and the goodness and skill of the doctors. I prayed to God also, even with my agnostic doubts about the true existence of such an awesome deity since that concept is so mysteriously suspect. Just look at how many millions of humans cannot agree on who and what "God" is, and what exactly are we supposed to believe. I ask myself, why couldn't "God" be more Godlike and straighten things out down here on the earth, his own grand plan, or at least give all his 'children' the same story line? The point is that you reach out to grab onto any seed of hope floating on the breeze and hang on to this 'lucky charm' with all your might. Yes, I might be able to believe in God if one of the miracles he performed would be to save my little daughter's life.

I cried with tremors of helplessness, usually in private, to not let my loved ones sense the depths of my pain; I told myself that" I needed to be strong". This was a promise made to myself then when my daughter was only twelve. These were the exact words that would come from my mouth this time, with my daughter now forty-five years of age and her life again in jeopardy.

When I met with the surgeon, Robert M. Stenz, D.O., after the post-surgery implant of the med port in her chest just above the right breast (which allows easy intravenous accessibility), he looked cautiously into my eyes and asked, "Do you understand what we're dealing with here?" With my voice trembling, I answered "I think so; and I need to be strong for my daughter" as tears blurred my vision and my thoughts and I couldn't speak other words. The surgeon touched my hand and said in a comforting voice, "The port implant surgery went very well. Let me know if I can answer any questions you may have". I thanked him and realized why my daughter felt such trust and liking for this doctor with the soft voice and caring eyes that seemed to be able to read my thoughts. Trust in your physician is so important. When I spoke about my brief conversation I had with the surgeon to Dede, she spoke the words she had held back saying out loud to me until now, "It's Stage IV". I felt a huge lump in my throat as I said, "Yes, but we have a great plan" (I meant we were all going to fight like hell to beat this thing).

In my perception, cancer had always been a mysterious, unwelcome stranger lurking in the shadows waiting to steal people away. My mother, who lived to be eighty-four, was burdened with many physical ailments and suffering, but she would repeat this phrase many times after a visit to the doctor, "Thank God, it's not cancer". In her young days, cancer was a dreaded curse because there was not effective treatment and many people suffered long and painfully with precious little hope.

The closest this "monster" called cancer had come to my private world is the fact that my paternal great-grandmother, Carrie Larson, died of breast cancer in the 1940's when I was not old enough to remember her; and my husband's mother, Hazel Arksey, died from breast and ovarian cancer in 1965. I knew Hazel only too briefly, but happily witnessed her joy at the thrill of seeing her grandchildren Dede and Dennis born before the advanced cancer stole her away from us.

Now cancer would not be such a stranger, but we wanted this unholy visitor to go away from our garden gate, far, far way.

***

DD:

When I first found out about our unwelcome visitor it felt like the rug had been pulled out from under me. My husband Ken and I cried together. We sat in stark, suffocating silence together, neither of us knowing what to say or do other than hold each other tightly. And we did. Tighter than we ever have, both afraid of what might happen to each of us during this season of our life together. But, resiliently, we agreed to take the positive approach. "This is just a bump in the road" we would say. But it hurt. And at first I felt mad; but I couldn't think of who I was mad at-so I got over that quickly and just decided I was going to fight. Like tender asparagus roots that lay dormant during the harsh, cold Michigan winters and then poke up through the earth every early spring, I decided that I would only let this experience toughen my roots during this particular "winter" of my life (even though it was sunny June).

My parents offered the same comfort and practical support they always have, confirming that we'd fight this together and that everything would work out. But I knew how much their world had been shaken when my daughter, Lindsay, called later that evening to say, "Grandma is 'freaking out', Mom. She just called and said I should call and tell you how much I love you. She was crying and everything!" After reassuring her that we would get through this (wondering to myself if I was lying to my baby) and hanging up the phone, my emotions overwhelmed me. I put myself in my mother's shoes and cried harder than I had yet, imagining what it would feel like if I ever heard this kind of news about my daughter. It is true that, as a mother, there is nothing that hurts more than if your child is hurting. Not even when you hear "stage IV breast cancer." I decided then and there I was NOT going to let this intruder take me away from my family.

The nights were the worst. I would wake up and all the "What if's" would invade my soul. I wilted a little. I clung to Ken in his sleep. I cried and whimpered. Then I would turn to God. Why was this happening? I asked for a miracle. I started being vigilant about watching Joyce Meyer on TV in the mornings when Ken left for work. I found I could see it at 8:00 a.m. if I missed the 6:30 a.m. show, and later found out I could even get it on the TV at 10:30 a.m. The messages uplifted my spirit and never failed to seem pertinent. I began to pray more calmly. And I turned my fate over to God. One particularly dark and lonely night, I suddenly felt like the sun had risen. I made a decision. I distinctly remember telling God, "I accept whatever you decide should happen. For my part I will go through this process with a positive attitude. I will try to learn as much as I can and have a faith that I can bear whatever ends up happening." I felt immediately lighter and calmer.

I took a new look at life. I wanted people to know how much they meant to me. I said "I love you" more frequently, even to some that I wasn't accustomed to saying it to. I hugged more freely. I smiled more readily. One particularly beautiful day while Ken and I were taking a group "ride" on our 2004 Harley Davidson, I became especially sentimental as my body swayed in unison with Ken's. As I snuggled up to his back, riding on the 'sweetheart seat', I squeezed Ken around the middle and told him, "I don't care if I have 100 years or 100 days as long as I can spend them with you"; and I knew in my heart of hearts that I meant it.

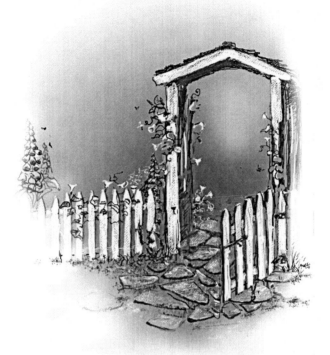

2

Discovering the
Garden of Being

MD:

These initial episodes in June and July 2006 would be the beginning of our exploration and discoveries into what I could describe as a walk into a vast garden where many new beautiful flowers and plants grow of all descriptions and sizes, from tiny sprouts to majestic trees that dwarfed every other growing thing. There were rocks, waterfalls, rolling hills, valleys and seas. There was challenge and beauty unlimited. This is how I began to view our earthly life. It was a feeling always felt inside me, but now it seemed to take on huge relevance. There were also dangerous twists, turns and drop-offs in this Garden of Being. Definitely, there were things to be avoided— poisonous things and predators who unpleasantly surprise the unsuspecting garden visitor. We would meet up with many other garden trekkers along the way, all sharing information on which direction to take to see the most wonderful attractions, as well as what to avoid. We were on a new journey.

A garden, to me, can represent a microcosm of a piece of the earth anywhere. A garden contains air, soil, water, both living and dying organisms, predators and prey. This can apply to a potted plant, also! Our body is like a garden, containing the same chemical earth elements. When we plant a garden, we often try very hard to make it perfect and balanced, filled with beauty, vigor, and abundance; but we soon find that it can easily get out-of-balance. It may be too weedy. It may be too buggy. It may be too wet or too dry. It may be tired out or trampled on. These are common results of neglect or abuse.

Our body is like a garden. It is subject to the same influences as a yard garden as it is composed of the same earth elements, oxygen and hydrogen (air and water), carbon, fluoride and several other common chemical elements.

Gardening is an art. It is not for the faint hearted. I learned this the hard way. My husband and I put in a good size garden shortly after our family of four (five counting our old dog, "Bones") moved to our five acre plot in Elba Township in Lapeer County in 1980. We wanted to taste a little of self-sufficiency and get close to Mother Nature and the Good Earth. Putting in the garden was an act of love. My husband, Richard did the hard work of tilling and digging out rocks. We enlisted the help of our son Dennis and his sister Dede to help with rock removal. They were not as thrilled about the garden project as mom and dad. Together we planted and watched as the seeds began to grow magically, along with a million weeds! Never having had much hands-on practice and getting our inspiration from books, especially the Mother Earth magazine, we found out quickly that a garden is a whole lot of work. There are a multitude of critters, tiny as a gnat and humongous as a deer, that love vegetable plants but oddly seem to ignore the weeds (some kind of conspiratorial relationship). We delighted in harvesting the vegetables (not many) that survived the bugs, weeds, raccoons and deer as well as our beginner's ignorance. We gained enormous respect for farmers and master gardeners that first season.

Growing and tending a successful garden is like taking care of our body to stay healthy, it takes proper preparation, the right combination of chemical composition and constant vigilance, and, if you are lucky, you will get the full cooperation of Mother Nature.

The biblical phrase, "As ye sow; so shall you reap" applies to both gardening and life. To me this means we live in a "Garden of Being". Life is a garden and it is lots of work, but the results can be extremely rewarding. When we choose to plant a garden, we should put honest effort and thought into the project from beginning to end. If we want to live a happy life inside a healthy body, we need to do the same.

Cancer in a human body destroying cells and tissues can be compared to leaf rot or plant blight in a garden. It can be deadly destructive. That is why you should take preventative actions such as annual examinations, healthy eating habits, and paying attention to suspicious bodily changes; and, if you or a loved one are dealing with cancer now; take all possible steps to remove all visible signs and remnants of the disease as you would if you discovered a destructive bug in your garden. As the garden responds favorably to the right weather, sun, rain and good gardening techniques, your body responds favorably to appropriate medical treatment enhanced positively by a healthy, healing specific diet, good mental attitude and many other alternative methods. This is what this book is about. It is to share our personal story of great discovery and success in The Garden of Being.

> *"Human beings, vegetables, or cosmic dust-we are all dancing to a mysterious tune, intoned in the distance by an invisible piper."—Albert Einstein*

In my childhood, my life garden was mostly weeds, with an occasional surprise of a flower bloom or chance encounter with wildflowers alongside a road. I did have a special "tree", a 20 ft maple that grew in my grandmother's front yard where I spent a good deal of my playtime. The tree was a retreat. When I climbed up and sat on the strong lower branches they felt like the loving arms of a faithful friend who waited for me to come out and play. My tree was a 'jungle gym', a playhouse and an observation tower. Sixty years later, I feel that this silver maple tree and I had much more in common than being made of a combination of the same earth chemical elements. We were both young, lonely, and stuck in one place having to make the best of it. In my case, I was dreaming of adventure finding me, as I did not have any concept of freedom at the time that I could venture very far from home. Maybe that is how my tree felt, too.

Richard (Rich), my husband for forty-six years at this writing, has made my life since our marriage a garden of sustenance and beauty. Our garden in the beginning consisted of nourishing each other with love and learning. Our garden "grew" two children, Denise (Dede) in 1961 and Dennis, three years later in 1964. The years of child rearing were committed to earning a living and the extent of our green gardening was maintaining a wooded lot and occasional patches of flowers. Richard's mother Hazel had tended and cherished a climbing red rose bush that clung tenaciously to a wooden fence at the front of the property. When we moved from this house to the five acres we have called home for the past twenty-six years, Richard dug up the rose bush and brought it with us. It has survived. He started new cuttings last summer with the goal of re-establishing this heritage rose bush at our children's homes. A memory of Grandmother Arksey will smile on us and her decedents from these sweet pinkish-red rose blooms.

Our senior years find us especially cognizant of our human connection with plant life. Rich has taken a great love for indoor plants (luckily our house has an interior sunroom/atrium ideal for plants) and outdoor plants and gardening in the summer. Our yard theme has an oriental, Japanese garden flavor. It is a labor of love that, due to Richard's muscle and effort, has long rock slab pathways, rock gardens and many decorative trees and shrubs that delight the eyes and senses. Being around live plant life is 'energizing' and healthy. Humans, through respiration, produce carbon dioxide, an essential component of plant life photosynthesis; and plants produce oxygen, a necessity of human life. It is a perfect partnership and a scientific fact.

I sometimes joke with friends that as a girl I dreamed of marrying rich. My dream came true; my husband is "Rich" and he has helped make my life garden to be filled with boundless devotion, love, playfulness. and a home that spells 'sanctuary'. A girl can't get richer than that.

***

DD:

"Your mind is a garden, your thoughts are the seeds; the harvest can be either flowers or weeds"—Author Unknown

We had all (me, Ken, my family and friends) entered into a new Garden of Being. Being was different now. Gone was the childlike ideal that our garden would automatically bloom the next season or the next, or the next. There was danger and we were looking it square in the face. I would have preferred to be a shrinking violet during this spring of my life, but I was not. I felt more like the ajuga plant, ugly and sickly looking in winter and early spring. Like the dormant ajuga patch sucks in water through it's withered, dry roots in the cold, damp ground, I took in all the information given at the oncologist's and surgeon's offices. I felt the love of my family and friends on my face like the warm, gentle rays of the sun on a bright sunny day. And I prayed to get better.

It was strange because I didn't feel sick. Oh, I had had more than my share of sick days in the previous few years. And hangovers were a norm for my social crowd. But the confusion of trying to reconcile this diagnosis with how I had been feeling physically just did not make sense. Could there have been a mistaken diagnosis? Was this really happening? I asked myself all the questions. But it was real and it was happening. My job now was to fix it.

So some immediate lifestyle changes were implemented. No alcohol. It was replaced with lots and lots of clean, "it's so-good-for-you" water. I began attempting to boost my immune system by taking 4life Transfer Factor®, daily. I started reading articles provided by my mom and others, as well as searching the internet for success stories and websites that provided information on the disease. This can quickly become overwhelming so I tried to limit those activities. And I, full force, practiced both visualization techniques and 'release' therapy by giving my situation over to God. And I felt comforted.

The other strong flowers I had chosen to share my garden with rallied around me. They protected me. They checked on me. They shared nutritional and nutritional supplement information with me. They let me lean on them. It was a variety garden. Using flower names for people personalities, there were dahlias, tulips, daisies, hollyhocks, pampas grass, roses, and more-each different but a great complement to the others.

When an obstinate and impolite "pumpkin plant" showed up trying to choke some of us out with its large, overbearing leaves, we weeded it out. My garden became my sanctuary. I, much later, identified how important this was to my health. Just one possibility of an encounter at the oncologist's office sent my blood pressure up and gave my nurse cause to ask "What is up with that?". My usual perfect blood pressure was high. To me, this was conclusive data that there are people, like incompatible plants, that just cannot share your Garden of Being—for your health.

Our garden was evolving into something it had never been before. Different focus. Different priorities. Different ideals. Different but not necessarily bad. I have practiced positive thinking for as far back as I can remember, but things were different now. The air was sweeter. Relationships became more rewarding. Finished projects became more fulfilling. Life became all encompassing. My Garden of Being was evolving, not dying. I planted that seed and nurtured it with everything I had.

> *John 15: I am the true Vine, and my Father is the Gardener. He lops off every branch that doesn't produce. And he prunes those branches that bear fruit for even larger crops.*

(This biblical rephrasing heard on Joyce Meyer TV show January 24, 2007)

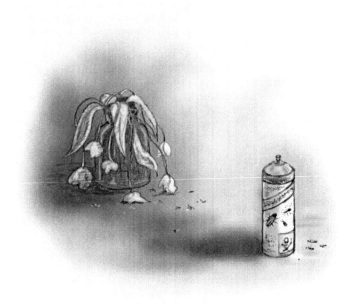

3

Chemotherapy
Bug & Weed Killer
for the Human Body

DD:

I came upon this analogy (and Chapter 3 title) during one of my "wanderings" through my backyard garden. I love flowers; I think it is something I inherited from my Grandma "T" (her nickname from grandchildren because "T" was shorter and sweeter than her last name, Troutt). We had found common ground on this subject as I grew up.

Every year brings new changes in our yard. Ken and I had completed many improvements in our backyard during the previous five years. Appropriately, some of the improvements had been funded by a small inheritance that had been passed down from my beloved Grandma T. We receive many compliments; and it is truly a beautiful view from my kitchen window. My garden had become my sanctuary.

I was walking down our sculptured cement pathway, spraying weed killer and trying hard not to hit anything deemed a "good plant", the budding poppy, balloon and sedum plants, when it hit me. Weed killer was just like chemo. We try to target the chemo drugs on the bad cancer cells, but some of the good cells end up casualties. The strong flowers only get a few "brown spots" but go on to flower and are beautiful season after season. The weak ones die. I, again, determined to myself that I would be a strong flower.

The first treatment of chemotherapy was the scariest. I guess it was fear of the unknown and "all that jazz".

The chemotherapy didn't turn out so bad. It helped that the nurses were knowledgeable, yet playful. Other patients who had been going through the process turned out to be priceless in the hope they give you when you are just starting out. Seeing someone who has been (in their words) 'baked, fried, cut and pumped' laugh and talk about how normal their life was is immeasurable to the psyche of a new chemo patient. I found myself thinking maybe this wouldn't be so bad after all.

As I lay back and tried to relax that first day of chemo, I DISTINCTLY heard an unfamiliar voice say "NOooooooo oooooooooooooooooooo-o-o-o-o-o-o". I looked around, it had sounded so real. And, even though I knew it had come out of my head, it wasn't me making the sound. And it wasn't God. I knew what God sounded like. I realized suddenly that it was the cancer. The cancer was melting from my body like the wicked witch of the west in the Wizard of Oz story when the munchkins doused her with a pail of water.

And so the treatments went. While you are on chemo, you are a member of a unique club. It's not a club you would volunteer for, but you are now a member nonetheless. As with all clubs, you have your unique language. Now conversations center around "What drugs are you getting?", "Did you have (pick from any of a dozen or more conditions) side effects?", or "How many times do you come for chemo?" and so on. The club and its members made the chemotherapy more tolerable and less frightening as we shared our every day human experiences.

I don't want to minimize the chemotherapy process. I tend to do that now that I am through the main treatment. Chemo was tough. There were bad days. I was a trooper, but chemo can zap your tap root.

***

MD:

Chemotherapy for Dede was begun as quickly as possible. It was June. There was no time to delay. There would be eight sessions spread out at two week intervals. These sessions would last from five to seven hours. It was helpful we lived only fifteen minutes apart and I could take an active role in being a co-caregiver as her husband, Ken, had to work. It was a necessity to keep bills paid, especially health insurance which was ever so critical now. The medical expenses would prove to be astronomical, but fortunately, insurance covered most. We had heard horror stories about other local people who had lost savings and even their homes to pay for cancer medical treatment. It is hard to comprehend that in the United States of America, super power of the world and with the finest in medical resources, that some of our citizens are not able to receive affordable life-saving cancer treatment. Why?

I quickly closed the door on my long real estate career, allowing myself full availability for when I was needed to help Dede and Ken. I had another mission now. My spirit was now "recharged" for my new assignment; and, most importantly, I felt needed and appreciated by those I loved so dearly. The greatest help I could give my child at this time was the gift of my time. It was only fair as she had always given me the gift of joy since the first time I held her in my arms. Jobs and marriage and babies would keep us living routines that somewhat pulled us in opposite directions for over twenty-five years. Now it was our turn to be closer than we had ever been before and to learn little things we had not yet discovered about each other as we both advanced into new levels of maturity. Most of all, we would learn the strength of our love. It made me feel proud to have my daughter invite me to be with her at doctor visits when Ken had to be at his workplace.

This new challenging assignment was very educational and eye-opening. It started with the first visit to the oncology specialist at the clinic in Lapeer, which by great fortune, is only ten minutes from her house. We had a big misconception that chemotherapy was a liquid medicine containing strong chemicals that a patient would drink (go ahead and laugh) and that it probably was the same "chemo cocktail" for all cancer patients. In fact, chemo is usually administered intravenously (and that was the purpose of the chest port implant), although some maintenance chemo is in pill form. Radiation and surgery of affected areas are other more radical treatment which was not recommended for Dede at this point. That was good news.

The first chemotherapy session was a frightening, but highly anticipated event. It would be the attack on the enemy! Dede and I packed snacks in a cooler in readiness for the possible eight hour session. The nurses were fantastic. One nurse sat down with Denise to explain the procedures and answer questions. A patient is weighed upon arrival, then blood is taken to check the red and white cell counts. Blood pressure rate and heart rate are taken to make certain the patient's vital signs are within an acceptable range to proceed with the treatment. There was a team of three nurse practitioners who were in constant motion, working in coordinated patterns, hooking up patients to their tubing, timing and recording each patient's dosages with clockwork precision. They set a timer to ring at a designated, estimated time each time a patient's chemo solution is started. This enables the process, which can involve one plastic bag of "magic potion" liquid or as many as seven or eight, to run smoothly and sequentially. The nurses gave each patient much individual attention, reinforcing medical advice and physician orders. We were impressed.

Some patients came in, snuggled into their big high top adjustable back chair and snoozed. Others shuffled in and some marched in. Dede danced in and brightened up the room immediately like a ringmaster at the circus who boldly and loudly announces, "Ladies and Gentlemen, Welcome to the Greatest Show on Earth"!

Dede was a livewire in the clinic chemo room, always joking with other patients and the nurses. She talked another patient, a sheriff deputy, into developing a new system of visually communicating with the nurses when they thought their chemo bag was ready for replacement by rolling the stanchion that holds the bags out in front of their chairs about a foot, sort of like a bar patron sliding their empty cocktail glass or beer bottle forward toward the bartender for a refill. It was hilarious to us, but I don't think the nurses thought it was quite <u>that</u> funny.

Most of the patients came to the clinic in jeans or sweat suits which makes sense because you want to be comfortable, but Dede turned each session into an occasion to wear something that would set her apart...a different wig or hat, business suit or fashionable casual wear along with coordinated jewelry. The nurses would 'gush' "Oh, don't you look great!" Comments like that do a lot for your mood. I think it also reinforces a theory about image. Dress like a bedraggled stray pup; that's how you'll likely feel. Dress <u>up</u> a little; feel <u>up</u> (maybe like a "Best of Breed show dog!)

It would be difficult to try to keep your identity or condition secret in the clinic environment unless you wore a disguise or made some advance and elaborate arrangements for private room treatment. Overall, the group setting seems to be very therapeutic. The patients did not seem at all self-conscious. There was a shared communion of hope; and except for a small percentage, the patients had ready smiles, high hopes and interesting stories to share.

I had decided to keep a journal record of treatment (dates, times, drug names and other observations) from start to finish. This kept me busy and involved and it turned out to be a very valuable reference for Dede to refer to and show to other doctors and clinic appointments. When someone asked what chemo was being given, they were grateful and impressed when shown a detailed, typed list, rather than getting a hazy and undependable oral recollection. Somewhere in my life I had been told to "Pay attention to details". In this case, I felt it was very good advice to put to use.

The chemo treatment did not cause Dede to have too many or severe side effects. There are several drugs administered to prevent nausea and counteract some of the damaging effects that chemo has on a healthy body. Some of these ancillary drugs included Aloxi®, Tagamet®, Decadron®, Benedryl®, and Heparin®. The powerful chemo drugs Dede received were Taxol®, Avastin®, and Adriamycin®, which cost as much or more than gold. Taxol® is made from the bark of the Western Juniper Yew tree usually found in the State of Oregon. We are harvesting (and copying) healing medicines from nature just like the American Indians did 200 or more years ago. Adriamycin® is highly potent man-made chemo drug. It is bright red in color; the only drug I saw that was not clear in color. It is nicknamed, "The Red Devil". The nurses were careful to warn that, "Don't worry if your urine is red afterwards; it's normal!" Yeh, I can imagine someone freaking out about red pee. That drug can adversely affect the heart activity, so it was discontinued for her treatment after six sessions because of her medical history and heart surgery.

After the second or third chemo, Dede felt like the wind had been knocked out of her. Until then, she had coped well. On one occasion, she had been scheduled for x-rays and had to fast that day and then drink four pints of barium liquid prior to the test. That was the scariest event, I think, related to her chemo. She was so nauseous and weak, we had to push her in a wheelchair to and from the test lab in the hospital. Ken and I waited in the visitor room at the hospital for Dede to return from the x-ray tests, I gave him a strong hug and tried valiantly to hold back tears. Sometimes the right words get stuck in our throats, so I knew the hug would tell him how much I loved him as a son-in-law and how fortunate I felt that my daughter had such a loving and devoted husband. He has a "Green Thumb" in the garden, too, besides many other wonderful talents.

That weakness passed quickly and the other most truly uncomfortable reactions were hot flashes. Chemotherapy can push a woman into early menopause, and it seemed to have that effect this time.

Chemotherapy is toxic, like bug and weed killer for the garden, but is designed to kill cancer cells that invade the body. Like any chemical pesticide, these drugs can have adverse side effects if not used with care. But, we are so lucky to have this powerful weapon to fight the disease.

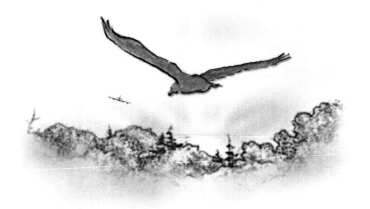

4

Flying to Discover
Hope and Promise

MD:

After her first four chemo sessions, Dede and I took an airplane flight to Cancer Treatment Center of America in Zion, Illinois, about 100 miles north of Chicago. We had read some positive reports and welcomed the opportunity that was presented to get a second opinion on the diagnosis and current treatment.

During the two days at CTCA, Dede was scheduled for scans, x-rays, and blood tests that went like clockwork. It was absolutely a world class operation just as the circulars had promoted. Every aspect of the center was impressive—the staff, doctors, and facilities. One of the most inspiring aspects about this visit was meeting some of the patient-clients who were from all over the United States and beyond (we heard people speaking what sounded like Dutch or German).

What had brought some patients to Zion, in addition to the advanced treatment programs, was that this was the only one in a chain of four CTCA centers across the United States that accepted their type of health insurance to cover treatment costs. That seemed very unfair to me. That meant that many, many people who did not have huge reserves of money might not get life saving cancer treatment.

We shared some of each category of laughter, tears, hope and encouragement with all of the patients we met. Each had unique personal cancer stories to tell. There was instant camaraderie.

The caregiver (patient's support person and trip escort) is given the highest courtesy in all respects, even being able to partake of cafeteria meals while at the facility and made to feel welcome and important in all instances. The staff members seem to recognize and truly appreciate the fact the people close to the patient play an important factor in the healing process.

We may have set a new world record for passengers in the shortest taxi ride ever taken (in Zion, Illinois, anyway). The second night in Zion we wanted to have a nice dinner at a recommended restaurant which happened to only be about the distance of barely a half city block from our motel. About the time we were heading out, planning to walk to the restaurant, a heavy rain began pounding down. Hungry and not to be deterred from our dinner plans, we decided to call a local cab service that advertised $5.00 fare anywhere in Zion city limits. The cab arrived and we hopped in. The cab started down the highway for about five seconds when we shouted, "There it is, stop right there!" The driver let out a shocked and unbelieving gasp, "HA, YOU ARE KIDDING, RIGHT?!" He dropped us off at the door, we paid the $5.00 fare and happily scurried into the restaurant, nice and dry. We laughed ourselves silly over our two minute taxi ride and how the taxi driver must have thought we were really a couple of weird women.

We returned home to Lapeer on the third day, both of us filled with confidence that the trip had been a good decision. The doctors there had supported the initial diagnosis and current treatment.

The biggest discovery was that the local treatment in Lapeer was not offering multi-discipline approaches to treatment as did CTCA where Dede had been counseled and introduced to nutrition and healing foods, naturopathy, spiritual support, pain management, mind-body-spirit, and emotional support treatment disciplines designed to treat the whole person in the healing process in addition to the medical remedies. There was a lot more to helping a person beat cancer than just taking the narrow path of conventional treatment. This discovery was awesome and inspiring. Chemotherapy may be the cancer bug killer in our garden of being, but there is so much more that makes a garden bloom and flourish!

There was a mind-set with all the facility staff at CTCA that gave encouragement of cure or improvement to each and every patient who was in need of hope. Cancer patients may want and need to "hear it straight" about the seriousness of their disease, but most want to hear that the doctor is willing to help and not to give up as long as the patient is willing to fight. Would it make our days on earth more or less precious if we could count them on a calendar? I think that we all should live each day as "if" it might be our last because we will treasure each second of each minute of each hour. Today is also the first day of the rest of our life! It's time to do good deeds, tiny or tremendous, that someone will remember us by to make our life count for something. We can start today!

During this trip to Cancer Treatment Center of America, Dede found more than hope, it was in the faces and smiles of everyone there—along with a promise—that if she needed to hear it, they were there to comfort, inspire and fight along side her in this battle. We heard with our own ears from several patients that they had been told by their doctor back home "to go and get their affairs in order". I know I don't want a doctor to give up before I do (maybe not even then)! Hope is a powerful treatment. No garden can grow to its fullest potential without it. A sturdy hoe, helping hands, a giving heart, and boundless hope are good partners in the garden.

DD:

Things were going well; as a flower I was holding my own. Everyone said I looked good; and as we know, "It is much better to look good than feel good, Dahling." Forgive me if I do my climbing rose impression and ride the fence on that one.

I was feeling better. I started to pursue the local hospital resource room for information, but was disappointed. I was told "eat whatever you want". Here I was looking for ways to help myself, and I got the impression that since I was stage IV, I was being pacified. Then I was mad.

From the minute I made my call to The Cancer Treatment Centers of America, I can honestly say I have never been treated with more dignity, compassion, and support from a medical facility. They are, hands down, the best of the best at what they do. The owners should be happy to hear that, in my experience, their goal to provide a facility that treats each patient with the same degree of care, the same care they would expect for their own mother, was met. Within forty-eight hours they agreed to see me and helped us locate accommodations at a local hotel. We were on our way and 'cultivating' my "Garden of Being".

Before we left, I received the PET (Positron Emission Tomography) results for a status after my first four rounds of chemo. It was encouraging! It seemed that there was no longer evidence of tumors on my lungs, liver or chest cavity. It was wonderful. But somewhere in the back of my mind, like the morning glory that droops when the clouds cover its all important sunlight; I was hesitant. As happy as I was, it was a surprise. Now more than ever, I wanted a second opinion. So Mom and I synchronized our wardrobe and made arrangements to fly to Zion, Illinois.

Everything went well at Zion. The nutritionist was fabulously helpful and gave me specific nutritional goals that were reasonable. Some things I had access to in my vegetable garden at home. We attended a group presentation to hear about their multi-disciplined approach to beating cancer which, along with medical treatment, included nutrition (top of the list), naturopathy, mind-body-spirit therapy, spiritual support and pain management. Mom and I attended a Qi Gong class, enjoyed and made notes about the variety of ultra-healthy food available in the cafeteria, walked the nature path along the small lake behind the hospital, and "kept the schedule" of tests I had received. And we laughed. It was a fun trip. Probably not what you would expect to hear from someone going for a second opinion on treatment for stage IV cancer, but it was. We had a strong blossoming week.

The verdict was good. The CTCA oncologist reviewed all the testing and told me that the chemotherapy I was receiving at home was the same regimen they would also recommend. We all agreed it made sense for me to not travel under the circumstances, and I returned home to continue with my "Round Up" treatments.

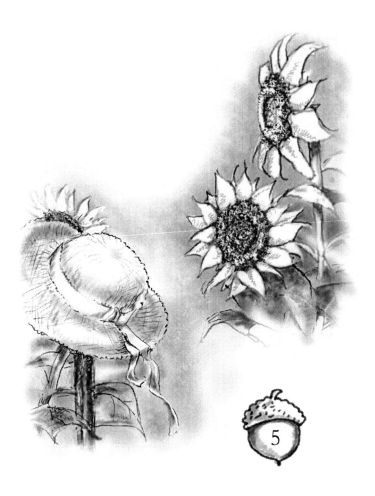

5

Buy a Garden Hat

DD:

It is true that I still say the worst thing that has happened to me during this summer of my life was losing my hair. It might have been even more traumatic if I had not had such a large support system. I guess watering my garden in the past helped sustain my spirit through the trauma of losing every single strand of hair on my head (including my eyebrows and eyelashes). I tried desperately to slow the process, wearing a bandana at night to hold my hair in place and not brushing, combing or touching it if possible. But all this effort only resulted in a hairy bandana wrapped around a detached "pony tail" of hair that I pretended (if I did not disturb it) was still growing out of my head! I made an appointment with my hair stylist friend, Jackie Smith, and she gently buzzed off the scattered patches that resembled clumps of brownish moss on a garden stone.

My father teased me, playfully, about now being eligible for membership in the Arksey men's 'Unhair club' of which he boasts he is the president. You see, both my brother, Dennis, and my dad have had clean shaven heads for many years. It looks good on them. In reminiscing over family photos it ALWAYS occurs to me that Dad looks younger today, at 66, with a bald head than he did at 30 with the 'horseshoe' hair-do. But, as a woman, I couldn't find it in myself to go "Bald and Beautiful". I felt more like I did at age fifteen when my dad first shaved his head. I was mortified. His head glowed white where there had been hair and now so did mine. When he first shaved his head, in 1977, no one voluntarily shaved their heads. That didn't become a trend until twenty years later. That first summer our family went on a month long tour of western America and everywhere we went people stared and quickly averted their eyes from ours. We always joked, "No, he doesn't have cancer". Now I did. And he has become, at least in his own mind, the fashion trendsetter of the times -for men. I didn't have what it takes to do it for myself or womankind. So................

I bought a stylish straw garden hat. Exposing my face and my skin to the sun was a "no-no" that I reluctantly accepted. And I really struggled with the wigs early on. One day I confided tearfully to one friend that "I just didn't feel like ME". But, like one particularly astute Radiation Oncologist shared with me during a clinic visit, it is amazing what we can actually adapt to when given enough time. Ken and I rode our motorcycle as much as we could. Our social group usually sported various degrees of 'helmet hair' anyway, so much of the summer was spent in "do rags" (bandana head wrap) and one particular cowgirl hat that my husband found especially appealing.

By September I was having fun with the wigs. My fall and winter ensemble planning now had to include:

***

1. Activity
2. Temperature (boiling hot flashes were becoming frequent)
3. What wig went with the "occasion"

***

My friends and I joked about alter egos for each wig, but I never really got that far. A rose is a rose is a rose in my Garden of Being.

***

MD:

It was a sure bet, Dede would lose her hair during chemo. No matter how much fun attitude and courage you try to muster, it is one of the more traumatic side effects for most patients, especially women. A family friend, Shelly McDonald, had a serious battle with cancer two years before and was a wonderful and supportive friend to Dede. From the very first day Shelly found Dede would have a similar experience with the big C, she gave Dede lots of tips to deal with the hair thing, including not being afraid of looking silly, but to concentrate on comfort, good times, good friends, and living. She also gave Dede something much more important. Shelly had survived and was going strong! Shelly was true inspiration.

Dede started "shopping" wig catalogs right away and picked out a couple that looked like they would be cute and not look too phony. She could turn this condition into her own fashion campaign. After a few months, she said, "Hey, Mom, it isn't so bad not having to wash, blow dry, curl and hairspray my hair every day!" In Michigan summers, a wig is like wearing a hat and your head will sweat. Dede solved this by wearing head scarves and cool straw hats. In winter, wigs serve as hair and hat combination and keep your head warm. Also, you can be mysterious and chameleon-like, showing up one day in a bouncy short hairdo, another day with a different color hair, or with long shoulder length sexy hair. You can pick your hair to fit your mood, like changing hats! You can have different wigs for your alter egos.

The young daughter of neighbors, Megan Jones, age 9, offered to cut her long hair, the color of corn silk, to make a wig for Dede. This was deeply touching. It was a tremendously loving and generous gesture from someone so young and whose heart was big for her size. Megan was a daisy in the garden, standing tall and glowing with sunny sweetness.

What's so important about hair"? Hair is like money; it's not important until you don't have any-if you want it. Some have written poems and prose about a maiden's hair. Oh, yes, there is the biblical story of Samson losing his strength when his hair was cut. There was a very famous Broadway play, Hair, and the other play and movie, Hairspray. But I think hair is overrated unless you are Godiva on her white horse and you don't have anything else to wear. Too much <u>ado</u> over a <u>hair-do.</u>

Hair is a little like the petals and leaves of plants and blooms which need constant attention and grooming to keep them at their most desirable state. Blooms need to be pinched off when they dry up and some plants respond with vigor when they are pruned and shaped. Cutting and grooming our hair is a little like grooming the leaves and vines of a plant. It is yet another trait we humans share with our gardens.

One of the funniest stories we heard about chemo hair loss came from a blonde haired, vivacious gal named Sherril we met at a Cancer Fighter's organization potluck meeting. She said that she had been absolutely certain that she would be one of the rare individuals who would not lose hair. She just knew it! She shared the following story with us.

On her way home from a trip to take her son back to college after his visit home, she was driving along with the window down, the warm late summer air rushing past and her Golden Retriever dog beside her. A wad of buff-colored hair floated past her and she grabbed it and tossed it out the window. Over the course of a few miles and the floating globs of hair getting thicker, she thought, <u>darn</u> it dog, why do you have to shed so much! The dog could not answer in people talk (and did not have to) because at that moment Sherril realized that it <u>wasn't</u> the dog's hair, it was hers! She laughed out loud and ran her fingers through her hair, feeling it detach itself from her scalp by bunches, and started tossing the strand bundles out the window to ride the wind like crepe paper party streamers. Half way home, she glanced in the mirror and said she looked like she had a scarecrow's head! She stopped at a small shopping mall that had ladies wear. The store clerk must have thought she had been in a cat fight or was drunk because when Sherril said defiantly, "I need a HAT", the clerk did not answer but, with an expressionless face and pursed lips, only extended her arm and silently pointed in the direction toward the hat display. We just about fell off our chairs laughing when we heard this story. Sherril was reliving the hilarious memory and was delighting in sharing her special comedy routine playback with us. I hope Sherril will appreciate that her story is bound to make many people laugh and feel good about poking fun at themselves, too.

Caution: Wearing wigs can be dangerous. Most are synthetic material as real hair wigs are very expensive, but both are flammable! On two or more occasions, Dede was leaning too close over their gas range in the kitchen and the front of her wigs were singed and crimped like fuzzy broken broom ends. It took a lot of trimming and tweaking to hide the damage. I would not recommend getting your wig close to any high heat or you may end up having a Michael Jackson experience, like when his hair caught on fire during a stage pyrotechnics display. If all else fails, you have to laugh at yourself, at least in between the tears. Whoever first said, "Bald is beautiful", must have been a Bald Eagle! The Bald Eagle is a proud, dignified and powerful bird with elegant beauty and a symbolic icon for the United State of America. But, it really isn't bald. It has feathers.

Dede's hair started growing back slowly about three weeks following her eighth chemo session. It was a great sign of progress, even though I'm sure she felt like a "Chia Pet", those clay figurines that you spread sprout seed paste on and watch it grow like a green grass fur coat. Luckily, her new hair wasn't green! It is reported that a person's hair might grow in entirely different than it was originally, maybe curly instead of straight or even a different color. This was not the case with Dede. Her natural hair was dark brown, slightly wavy, and fine in texture. I told her it reminded me again of when she was a baby with peach fuzz for hair, like a precious rosebud not yet in bloom in our "Garden of Being".

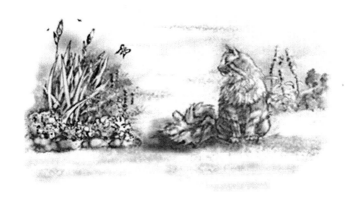

6

Get a Garden Cat

DD:

I have a cat who acts like a dog. No kidding. Her name is B.C. which stands for Birthday Cat. She was named for her unlikely arrival day. We were having a birthday party for my daughter, Lindsay, when she arrived. She was a straggly, stray puff of fur with the biggest orange tail you've ever seen. She had the sweetest little face and wasn't afraid of us at all. Rather she seemed to crave having us touch and pet her, an experience that seemed new to her. It may have been a new treatment, but she knew she liked it. It was heartbreaking to see something so tiny, one of God's gentle creatures, so neglected. I think I loved her from the first moment I laid eyes on her, just like her new 'sister', my beautiful Lindsay. Ironically, as I rolled history over in my head, it was actually seventeen years to the day I had brought Lindsay home from the hospital to this very house.

A cat is a perfect pet to keep you company when you are undergoing cancer treatment. Cats love long naps and staying warm. They see you the same no matter what hat or hair you are wearing-or not wearing.

B.C. comforted me when I felt bad and played with me when I felt well. She, too, loved our backyard garden and there were days when after countless (and frustrating to me) trips in and out, B.C. would lure me to the back door and then refuse to come in as if to say, "Come out and play!". Her favorite game is "ambush" which earned her one of her many nicknames, Ambush Cat. B.C. would 'ambush' you from the hall as you left the bathroom or jet across our backyards (ours and the neighbors) to playfully bat your legs as if to say, "Na-na-na-na na, Gotcha!" and then dart off out of reach. One of the funniest examples was when our neighbor, Julie Jones, was weeding her garden and was scared out of her wits when something soft all of a sudden grabbed a hold of her leg. Quickly, she realized it was B.C. and had to laugh. Ambush Cat would get all of us at one time or another.

Not all of her habits were loveable though. No one was too happy when she took to using the Jones kids' sandbox as her personal litter box. Worst of all, their dog, Casey, acted as a canine pooper scooper, eating the sandy "presents". This prompted Lauren Jones, age six, to ask me to "Please have a talk with B.C. and make her stop doing that." I told her I would, but that I wasn't sure she would listen.

So B.C. wasn't always a good girl, but she was my perfect pet. She would snuggle with me even when I didn't feel good enough to actually go out to the garden with her. There were days that all I had the energy for was feeding myself and B.C. She embraced my new healthy eating style, too. As I drank my morning liquid yogurt, she would purr up close to me and sniff at the container. After awhile it became part of our morning ritual for me to pour her a tablespoon full on a plate to share the breakfast treat.

After we received the test results which showed me in remission, I began to believe that B.C. had been our "test". We had passed. We had found it in our hearts to take her in, get her medical treatment (including being spayed), love, protect and nurture her back to health. And God had found it in his power to do the same for me.

A cat doesn't see you as a flower in your garden but rather the sun in theirs. Watch for a future book all about B.C. She <u>is</u> that funny.

***

MD:

B.C. the cat is a success story. When I first saw her, she looked so horribly pitiful-skin and bones, weepy and infected eyes, matted and stringy fur. But this "bag of bones" cat had certain sweetness; and the squinty alley cat eyes seemed to say, "Please help me". Dede saw a creature in need and set about to feed and clean her up. In typical mother fashion, I warned Dede, "That cat might have a serious disease". It was too late. Dede's adoption of B.C. (the Birthday Cat) was official. No turning back. It took two or three months of their trips to the vet, healthy cat food diet (catnip for diet supplement) and observation, but I think the most important element of this cat rescue and recovery operation was *love*. Love is given. Love is returned. B.C.'s love is a special nourishment to Dede's garden of being. B.C. started looking great-bright eyed, full of energy and she blossomed (like a spring dandelion with a fluffy coat of yellow-gold colored fur). B.C.'s initials now could be for Beautiful Cat!

A cat is especially designed to be a good garden pet because they tread so lightly around the plant life, rarely digging unsightly holes (except for fluffing up some dirt to cover some dainty feline feces). Cats are fun to watch chasing butterflies, bees and dragonflies. But there are other garden pet choices.

A dog, if kept under a watchful eye, can be an extraordinary garden buddy. My dog, Babe (a buff colored Labrador mix breed) loves to watch my husband and me work in the garden and yard. A dog knows exercise is <u>good</u> <u>for</u> <u>us</u>. She tags along every inch of the way, pausing to sit or lay and panting happily, when we stop to engage in the serious work of digging, planting, pruning, or harvesting. She may be helping in many more ways than a dog can contemplate. Babe helps by lifting my spirit with her loving eyes, waggy tail and bouncy gait. At eight years old, Babe has almost caught up with me in 'dog years' and would be considered a canine senior citizen. I try to act as energetic as she to prove I can keep up with her (we both, however, sleep much more these days and take longer breaks).

A dog makes us feel good about ourselves by providing affirmation of our importance (at least to them). The following says it so well:

"I want to be the kind of person my dog thinks I am"—
Anonymous

A dog or cat is not judgmental about our appearance, our bank account or our social status. This unconditional affection is therapeutic and healing to the human spirit.

I don't believe organic gardeners would endorse untreated dog manure as good fertilizer, but this is a true story. My mother and stepfather kept two large Doberman dogs in a 12'x 12' pen in the corner of their yard for about two or three years. The ground in the pen was layered with straw periodically and cleaned on an 'erratic' schedule, so it could be said the ground became highly 'enriched' with dog droppings over this time period. The dogs were sold and the pen was dismantled. The following summer my parents tilled this corner of the backyard and planted tomatoes. The tomato plants grew like Jack's magic beanstalk, reaching five feet tall and the tomatoes were as big as grapefruits! If I recall, the tomatoes were delicious, although I may have enjoyed them more if I didn't know where they were grown. Yuck!

This past fall, I spent two hours planting and staging a tulip flower bed, meticulously laying out the bulbs in a precise, well thought out pattern. When the bulbs were tenderly planted, I gently patted the cool soil on top as if tucking a blanket around a child at bedtime. The next morning, I glanced toward the tulip bed, imagining how glorious it would look next May. There were whitish blobs scattered over the freshly turned soil about the size of golf balls. Oh, No! It couldn't be the tulip bulbs! But taking a closer look, I saw that it WAS the tulip bulbs. Our dog Babe (or the neighbor dog—or a raccoon?) had been after a mole who may have been after white grubs which are plentiful in our yard. I took a deep breath and began resetting the two dozen tulip bulbs. When I finished, I placed a grate from a barbeque grill over the buried bulbs and covered the entire flower bed with landscape ground cover material, securing the edges with rock weights. I figure if my dog was the culprit, she was teaching me to be more creative and defensive in my gardening skills.

A dog can create a nuisance in the garden if distracted by a mole, mouse or rabbit. Your dog will think it is only helping you by keeping uninvited creatures away from the garden when, in the chase, plants get knocked down and holes get dug. Be forgiving. We humans often also create 'collateral' damage in our life unintentionally. Holes can be filled and plants replanted. Friendship and loyalty are worth the extra effort.

If you prefer a lower maintenance garden buddy than either a dog or cat, consider a frog. A frog can eat harmful insects. A frog looks good in the garden setting and most often blends in and is hardly noticeable at all. Frogs don't cost much to feed. You don't need to hire a frog-sitter if your frog lives in the garden. A frog is quiet (usually). However, a frog is not cuddly and not inclined to lick your face at the exact moment you may feel like you need a 'kiss'. There is, however, the story about a kiss turning a frog into a prince (in case you want to try). Pets, like people, have their good and bad points. Some are warm and fuzzy; some are cool and clammy, and some have warts. Brr-r-r-p-p.

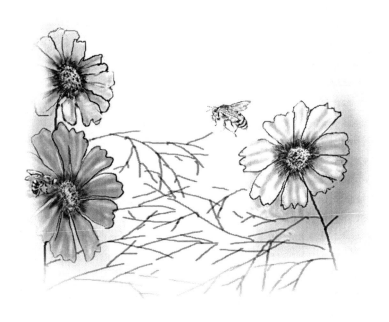

7

A Good Garden Takes
More Than Luck

MD:

This chapter reflects on mindset and how attitude impacts the healing process and life in general. The attitude referred to is not only the patient's attitude about their disease, but the attitude of others in the family (and also the acquaintance section) of their "Garden of Being". Using the garden analogy, weeds spread by sinisterly creeping and placing a stranglehold on healthy plants. If you want to flourish and be a glorious rose bush, tomato plant, or even a majestic oak tree, you need to grow away from the harm of choking weeds. You need accessibility to sunshine, air, water and essential nutrients— just like a plant or tree. You need to associate with people with positive, nurturing attitudes who provide the essentials for a healing atmosphere. Avoid people with negative or disruptive personalities (the WEED PEOPLE) whose attitudes attempt to choke out life-affirming spirit. I believe, with much pride, that our family and Dede's friends united in the common goal of providing the fullest measure of positive attitude and support to help her retain her strength and be a brilliantly blooming flower in her Garden of Being.

After the eighth chemo session in November 2006, a PET (Positron Emission Tomography) scan was scheduled to measure progress of treatment for Dede. REMISSION! Our family was elated to hear that no visible tumors could be found. It was a miracle! Our holidays over Thanksgiving, Christmas and New Years were fantastic. Dede was full of energy and ideas. She was able to give support to our other daughter (in-law), our lovable Cindy who was going to have abdominal surgery just four weeks before Christmas. She knew there was a tumor and that this surgery would involve exploratory methods. We were all praying for Cindy and praying that cancer would not have the audacity to strike again in our family circle. We received more good news following Cindy's surgery. No cancer! This was going to be a truly wonderful Christmas for our family.

Dede and Cindy were responsible for promoting a handmade gift exchange for Christmas 2006. Incomes were down and it seemed like a very good idea. At first, I felt a little panic, wondering what I could "hand craft"; I was out of practice for stuff like that. But the efforts and results were phenomenal. Cindy hand crocheted fluffy yarn neck scarves, even letting us pick our own colors. Dennis, my son, made wood plant stands of his own design for me and my husband and personalized wood-burned wall signs for the guys. Dede made sentimental holiday wall décor items using lace doilies made by her Great-Grandmother and selected favorite books from her collection to re-gift to each family member accompanied by a sweet personal message. I managed to think of something to hand make with my husband's assistance. These were three foot high grapevine holiday décor trees (grapevines were grown on our property) and scrapbooks (purchased) with a starting photo page collage for each person's scrapbook also containing a special original and personalized poem. Ken and Dede assembled small sacks of all the ingredients for a Kenny's Famous spaghetti dinner—homemade sauce, bag of noodles and a fresh baked loaf of bread. I was proud beyond measure of the creativity and love I knew went into all the gifts. Michael, our grandson, made wood turned casing ball point pens for the men and an art quality wooden trinket holder for his Dad. Lindsay, our granddaughter, presented hand baked Christmas cookies and seasoned snack mix bags all decorated with bows. It was the best Christmas ever.

We all agreed to try to do the handmade gift exchange again the next year. It would begin a new tradition. We already had sort of a "save the prettiest bows and boxes" to recycle year to year as long as they lasted. It was like a game and it was fun to try to remember "who gave who what" wrapped in the familiar decoration and carried over good memories of Christmases past to the next.

Our wonderful holiday celebration that year made me so aware that the Garden of Being takes so much more than luck. All of the gifts exchanged that were made by hands and hearts made me realize that love makes the Garden of Being beautiful beyond words.

***

DD:

I have always taken pride in being lucky. I had wholeheartedly agreed with many an associate who had made the statement "It is better to be lucky than good". Ken reminded me, even now, that I am the luckiest person he knows. Still somehow, this season didn't seem to be the time to rely on luck alone. So I researched. I read every article I saw or my mother found on cancer. I surfed the internet looking for success stories. I wanted to sow my seeds and have a fruitful harvest. I took all the input and put together a plan of action.

It's a little harder than finding ordinary garden manuals because, let's face it, there are not many "successful gardening" books out there about beating cancer. There are some; and I found more the longer I looked; but unfortunately, most of us just "go along" with whatever the doctors tell us. My community lacked in the area of ancillary cancer care. Besides, anyone going through cancer hears over and over, everyone is different. So even if I was a Lily-of-the-Valley, which is said to bring good luck but is also prone to host snails and slugs which eat holes in their leaves, there were no guarantees that my choice of commercial snail and slug bait would eliminate my body's "snails and slugs".

As it turned out, I had been doing some very good things for myself from the very beginning. I started drinking lots of purified or spring bottled water and taking a nutritional supplement, 4life Transfer Factor®, as soon as I was diagnosed. A very good friend, Dick Zahoranski, had colon cancer in 2000 and had beaten it. At first I think I took it just because I was so scared about the side effects of the chemo. The testimonial about others who had taken it and insisted it eliminated or helped to avoid side effects made me want to take it just to avoid the discomfort I was reading about. It turned out to be so much more as I learned through reading and confirmed at CTCA. This supplement was boosting my immune system to help it eliminate the cancer cells in my body and fight the side effects of my chemo treatments.

After we returned from CTCA, I started looking for other ways to help myself. I experimented with new menus, eliminated white bread, pasta, soda pop, alcohol, and anything I thought of as "processed". "Good bye, Hamburger Helper-it was a great relationship, but we've grown apart". Mom and I had fun planning and telling each other about our healthy meal of the day. I scolded my nurses for ordering fast food and shared yummy recipes with other patients and friends.

I know my extra efforts helped. And it occurred to me that in the past I had expected miracles of my body. Like the lovely Flowering Cherry tree, your body can be crippled by too much or not enough fertilizer, water or sun. Fungi can attach to wound or kill this delicate tree the same as cancer can do to the human body. In addition, conditions of heavy traffic or smog can require extra care for both this delicate tree and humans.

I boosted my immune system with Transfer Factor®, had my bottled water tested to confirm purity and changed my eating habits in order to 'stack the deck' and not solely rely on the luck that had gotten me this far. And I flourished.

My sister-in-laws were some of my flowers with healing influence. Ken's three sisters, Barbara, Nancy and Betty Jo, each helped in their own special way. Barbara, whom I like to think of as our family 'Peony' had a beautiful plant sent to cheer me at one of my lowest moments in treatment; this plant is still flourishing in the entry way of our home. Nancy, our cheerful family 'Daffodil', who is also a pharmacy technician, called to check on me after each treatment. She wanted to verify that I was getting all the right information about the chemotherapy I was receiving, the importance of regular water intake and how to combat side effects. Betty Jo, the exotic Hammerberg 'Hibiscus', sent me the cutest Anne Geddes cards 'darn near' weekly throughout my treatments to help keep my spirits high and my attitude positive. My brother's wife, Cindy, our colorful, flashy and vibrant petunia, was involved in bringing me treats and smiles in the evenings after her busy work day.

But the flower of honor, our pretty pink bloom climbing rosebush, was my mother, Dolly. Hardy enough to bloom profusely, but tender enough to require a support foundation of family to cling tightly to, she was my ever ready advocate. Nothing could come between her being with me at treatments or ensuring I had everything I needed in the days after treatment. She seemed to intuitively know just what I needed when, even when that meant letting me have time alone.

Luck is a wonderful thing to have in your corner, but you cannot rely on luck alone. You have to tap into all your resources—medicine, supplements, nutrition, love and faith to bring your "Garden of Being" to maximum blooming condition.

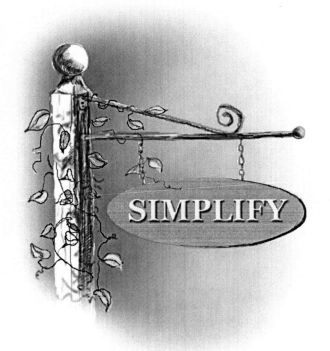

8

Simplify

MD:

This was the year in my life I adopted the theme, "simplify." To me this means being able to draw upon the resources close at hand or within, to reuse, recycle and respect things we already have, especially the good gifts of nature which we should also revere. This theme seemed to fit perfectly with our "Garden of Being" mindset.

"Live simply, so others may simply live"—Gandhi

Over the years my life had accumulated so much useless "stuff" it was nuts. I would stand in my closet looking at all the clothes "I just *had* to have" and not be able to think straight. It would take me way too long to decide what to wear. What a waste of time! I tried (and am still trying) to throw out "stuff" that I've had around for twenty years or longer and will likely never use in another twenty years. Maybe I'm trying to "trick" my brain or fool myself, but I feel that it was a very positive action to clear off the top of my computer deck hutch and put one single item there, a wooden sign that reads, "S-i-m-p-l-i-f-y" in six-inch high silhouette letters. It stares me in the face every day and I must try to obey.

Simplify, to me, means to center on the most important aspect in our lives and not let that get covered up by a lot of other "stuff", job-related worries, "keeping up with the Joneses", and buying "stuff" we don't need. It feels so liberating.

My attitude toward money included the belief that shopping was "therapy". No more (well, maybe just a <u>little</u> now and then). Attitude is the key word. It is true that money, like hair, doesn't matter unless you don't have any. Money is a tool, not something as inherently useful as a loaf of bread or a gallon of milk. Attitude toward money is healthy if its value is measured according to needs. If you measure your goal for money or material objects according to desire alone, enough is never enough.

"Too many people spend money they have not earned,
to buy things they don't want, to impress people they
don't like".—Will Rogers

On the subject of getting rid of clutter and putting some simplicity into your life, think of this. A house cluttered with unused, unnecessary, and unappreciated "things" is like a garden that is overgrown with undesirable, choking weeds and root bound plants. When this happens, the optimum beauty and growing conditions are lost.

Simplifying our life can make us healthier emotionally, I'm convinced; and it has to have a positive impact on our health when we get sick or encounter a disease like cancer. What might appear at first glance to be very simple, to reach out or be ready to embrace emotional support from friends and loved ones is the most powerful and effective medicine you can take.

When I saw the following quote by Albert Einstein, who is one of my historical idols, I thought to myself, this is great! Einstein supposedly professed to be an agnostic, like me, but he, too, sometimes invoked the name "God" when there did not seem to be any other answer. Other scientists have called it Einsteinian religion (Einstein did not profess to believe in God, but used the word for some unnamed and unknown control mechanism in the universe). I felt Albert and I had a connection!

"When the solution is simple, God is answering." Albert
Einstein

It seems everything in our society is becoming too complicated. For example, choices of products in the grocery store. I can remember about forty years ago we had about six different cereal brands to choose from; now there are about fifty and not all are high in nutritional value. I used to be able to name the make of any car driving down the highway; now I can only recognize maybe a half dozen out of fifty or more. The same applies to make up products, liquid refreshment, candy bars, cold medicines, pet food and pain relievers. Although I enjoy variety and choice, it scrambles my mind and stresses me out, making me want some of those extra-strength pain relievers (of which we have a dozen or more to choose from-giving me an even bigger headache).

My daughter and I are continuing to work on the simplicity theme in life—each inspiring the other at every opportunity. She sent me the following message found on an internet motivational site:

> *Many people believe simplicity implies doing without.*
> *On the contrary.*
> *True simplicity is both buoyant & bountiful, able to*
> *liberate depressed spirits from bondage and burden of*
> *extravagance and excess.—anonymous*

Webster's Dictionary includes part of the definition for simplicity as "uncomplex", "absence of cunning or deceit", "sincerity" and "good sense".

Simplicity means focusing on what really matters in our Garden of Being.

What really *matters?*

- It doesn't *matter* how big a house you live in.

<u>A house needs to be just big enough to hold enough love.</u>

- It doesn't *matter* what year or model car you drive.
  <u>A car that runs well is nice.</u>
- It's not the size of a person's bank account that *matters.*
  <u>A *personal assets account*-honor, humor, love, and trustworthiness is priceless.</u>
- "*Matter*" is just a conglomeration of molecules into assorted shapes.
  <u>A *"matter"* of opinion is usually always subject to scrutiny or exception.</u>

To be content with little is hard; to be content with much, impossible.—

Marie Von Ebner-Eschenbach.

***

DD:

Somewhere around my ninth or tenth chemo therapy most of the side effects were very minimal. Some hot, hot, HOT flashes, and a nap here and there, but for the most part I was feeling more normal than I had since the first treatment.

Simplifying took the form of cleaning and organizing every nook and cranny of our home. Closets were torn apart with a frenzy, kitchen cupboard interiors were fashionably papered to coordinate with our kitchen décor and made more "user friendly". My husband asked, "Why have a potato chip cupboard that never has potato chips in it?" This was a testimonial to our newly embraced eating habits.

"Where we were specialists in spending, we are becoming specialists in living."—Author Unknown

I've always loved being able to do something new with old treasures and I threw myself into my projects with a passion. Instead of buying new things, I recycled, reused and rejuvenated possessions we already had at hand.

Everything I did turned into an organizing adventure. A search for the James Taylor CD could turn into the whole CD collection being alphabetized. Creating my weekly grocery list could result in a couple of cupboard shelves being 'reorganized' so I knew what we already had in reserve—I think you get the idea!

Christmas gifts were made from family heirlooms, hand-me-downs and things I no longer had a specific use for. My home 'office' was FINALLY shaping up with new window valances (made from material purchased 15 years ago to make a bathrobe for Ken), hauling a long forgotten chair up from the basement, and even longer forgotten crocheted treasures from my ancestors.

The basement was becoming, rather than the scary, embarrassing place it used to be, into an organized combination of functional storage place and laundry room. You could actually start to see where a new bathroom **could** at least be installed when we pulled together the funds.

And it struck me, once again, that we are always, like a garden, in a perpetual state of change. Our leaves fall, our soil sometimes gets frozen over, but we are still there, ever changing, surviving and holding out for the warmth of the sun on our face.

And life felt good.

***

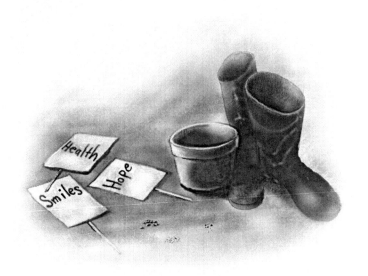

Seeds for Success

MD:

Dede and I read everything we could get our hands on about cancer cures and treatment. Common sense advice included things like:

- Do not drink alcohol during chemotherapy and don't drink to excess anytime if you want to be healthy (sober and sane I might add).

- Stay out of direct sun during chemotherapy as skin is ultra sensitive.

The chemo treatments gave Dede's skin a reddish flush much like a light sun burn. Too much sun can cause skin cancer and there is no dispute within the medical community about that. There are topical lotions that do a good job of "fake bake" on skin. Tanning booths, in my opinion, are torture chambers.

- Vitamins and anti-oxidant foods that claim to prevent or help cure cancer became our quest. Dede was careful to check with her doctor on use of vitamins and supplements.

- Aerosol sprays contain hydro-carbons and breathing these vapors are BAD for you and the atmosphere. Spritz sprayers are more environmentally friendly.

- I decided to replace my stick deodorants with those that did not contain aluminum salts. These can be found at health/natural food stores. One I like very much is Avalon Organics® herbal based deodorants.

- Most toothpaste brands have ridiculous ingredients, including lots of dyes. I switched to Tom's of Maine® toothpaste which is formulated with natural ingredients. It is <u>white</u> with no color dye (makes sense to me since tooth enamel is <u>white</u>—not red, green or blue like some toothpaste).

***

For so long we had been blissfully ignoring good eating and health habits. Our body "gardens" can become garbage trash receptacles. It was time to turn over a new leaf!

This is mainly a fun observation, and just an introduction to healing foods. Many (not all) of the very best anti-cancer and healthiest foods start with the letters **A-B-C**:

A-Apples, asparagus, artichoke, apricots

B-Broccoli, blueberries, bananas, barley, Brussels sprouts

C-Cabbage, cauliflower, cherries, citrus, carrots and chocolate!? (<u>dark </u>chocolate that is-not a true top-of-the-list health food, but consider it a not-too-dangerous treat in small bits as it actually has good stuff in it).

There are many more covering most all the alphabet A—Z. It was a new life resolution-eat to live; don't live to eat! Cookbooks for healthy living were like sexy novels; I could not get enough.

The safety of our food supply is at great risk. Commercial prosperity for food producers and distributors has resulted in people-poisoning all too often. For years and years, food manufacturers advertise products as "new", "improved", "enriched" and more "flavorful". Consumers buy these claims "hook, line and sinker".

Our foods are so adulterated with indigestible, sometimes harmful ingredients with zero nutritional value, it is no wonder Americans are overweight, yet undernourished, and plagued with many health-related ailments. Many people are "snack happy" and think that as long as they are stuffing something into their mouths, it's a good thing; but it is a dangerous habit. It is us, the consumers, who are primarily to blame for not insisting on safer standards and for continually buying inferior food products just because they are advertised in fancy commercials. The trend toward organic foods is a good omen. We can "vote" with our dollars.

Phytonutrients are elements naturally produced by plants or existing in the earth. Phyto is a Greek word for "plant". Phytonutrients include vitamins, minerals and enzymes essential for a healthy body. Most food supplement manufacturers derive their products directly from nature, but in the process, they lose most of the beneficial essence of the original plant. That is the reason you can derive much more benefit from eating natural, unprocessed food.

Rachel Carson's "Silent Spring" is an essential reading for serious environmentalists. In this prophetic book published in the early 1960's, she exposes the dangerous proliferation of "biocides" (herbicides and pesticides) as "elixirs" of death, along with hundreds of industrial chemicals, inorganic cleaning compounds and fertilizers. The production and use of these "elixirs" of death have been increasing at a seemingly unstoppable speed for the last fifty or more years. They permeate every corner and aspect of our earth and its inhabitants (that includes us, folks). The biological fall-out is believed by many scientists to cause malignancies. This may be why cancer is the number one killer disease in the U.S.

You might ask, don't we have a say in all this? We do. But only we speak out and only if we stop buying and using every 'ding-dang' new death spray-in-a-can that comes on the market. Global pollution is a massive problem that should worry everyone.

Euell Gibbons was a media celebrity in the 1960's who advocated eating natural foods found in the wild. He wrote a book called, "Stalking the Wild Asparagus". People poked fun of him as an eccentric, but he had a great idea at the time. However, these days you would want to think twice about picking wild asparagus or mushrooms along a dirt road, in a country field or in a forest as they may have been sprayed with toxic weed or insect killer. Chemical spraying has been done too indiscriminately, without thought or planning for the unfortunate repercussions to human health.

Chemical and drug companies provide the big bucks for the majority of research grants at colleges. This enables (almost insures) the results will be obligatorily in favor of the companies' products, not in the primary interest of human and environmental health.

"We must change our philosophy, abandon our attitude of human superiority and admit that in many cases in natural environments we find ways and means of limiting populations of organisms in a more economical way than we can do it ourselves".
- Canadian entomologist G. C. Ullyett

Biological balance is nature's proven formula; however, the biological way to control insects has a serious foe which is corporate profits. The reason is because the smell of money is as irresistible to most humans as a natural chemical pheromone is to a fly.

Slivers of radiant light are beginning to shine through "cracks in the door". This door opens to a hypothetical laboratory where solutions to earth's toxic pollution are discovered and implemented as the 21st century inches forward. There are activists, groups and (a precious few) corporations who are working hard for a clean and safe environment and biological balance in our world. Unfortunately, national governments (including the United States) are not the strong force they should be in leading the campaign for a healthy earth.

We have undeniable global warming and global pollution. Our earth garden needs overdue attention, respect and tender loving care. Visit this web site www.greenpeace.com.

"We are not passengers on this planet earth; we are the crew."—Marshall McLuhan

Listen to your doctors (some of them are very smart), investigate cancer treatment options on your own, listen to friends (they mean well) and sift through all these seeds of possibility and select those that you feel can help you grow your "Garden of Being" to its fullest potential.

There are many great books and magazines that contain great advice and menus for good nutrition. By eating healthy, you are planting seeds of success for your own body's healthiest Garden of Being.

***

DD:

I knew now that what I wanted to do with my life was different than how I had previously measured success. There was no way I was going back to a sixty hour per week job trying to get automotive parts delivered where they should be; it seemed so trivial at this point.

I began to try my hand at supporting other cancer patients in the community by reaching out to them as they were starting the cancer fight. I assembled folders to hold medical information, calendars, CTCA literature; and sometimes, a small polished gemstone or rock for them to hold on to during treatments or other rough times. I felt like, in some small way, that I was for a brief moment their gardener, watering gently, mulching around the vulnerable spots, and providing the warmth of encouragement.

The basic, consistent message I send out to anyone who is working to eliminate cancer from their garden is:

1. Drink lots of clean, safe water.
2. Eat healthy (avoid processed, fatty food).
3. Take a multi-vitamin daily
4. Investigate immune boosting supplements. I used Transfer Factor, a 4life® product, but be sure to discuss ANY supplement with your doctor. Understand that, usually, they won't endorse anything outside of their prescribed 'protocol'. Your job is to ensure nothing you take will interfere or adversely react with your medical treatments.
5. Believe in yourself and visualize eliminating cancer from your body.
6. Exercise and be active as much as is comfortable.
7. Get a second opinion—even if you like your doctor.
8. Contact me anytime—I'll be there for you.

The all encompassing message being that the foundation of a bountiful garden was having healthy, fertile soil that was organically enriched and watered. And it was great, and I knew I was making positive change. But I needed more. I needed to help more and on a larger scale.

It was at this time that I came upon an idea to utilize the management skills I had acquired the last 25 years along with my now identified status as "career patient". I put together a proposal for my oncologist on complementary and alternative cancer initiatives, wrote a letter to the newly appointed director of oncology at the Great Lakes Cancer Institute-McLaren campus, received water baptism, and began writing this book. Not only did I now have a direction; I was headed in the right direction. It would make sense why this happened to me if somehow, in some way, other people would benefit from my experience and success. I knew where I wanted to go and was sure I knew how to get there.

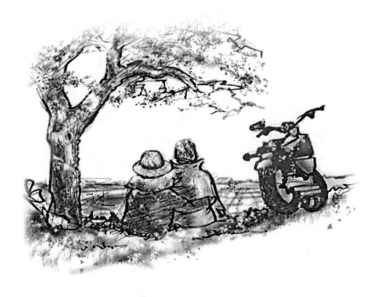

10

Laughter is Music
in the Garden

DD: Laughter and music truly were the two social "sports" we played during 2006. Money was tight now that we were living on one income and entertainment needed to be more than economical. It helped that we had so many close neighbors and the phone, along with email, helped me stay in touch with those that weren't planted quite so close.

There was only one rule for our garage (the neighborhood hang-out), "No crying at the Red Eye Inn" (official name for our garage 'Rec' room). And we never broke this rule.

Music, sometimes referred to as the "universal language", played a big part in our lives, as always. Ken was usually our DJ, picking his favorite songs and polling the group for theirs', spinning tunes to keep all of us singing and dancing.

There were a couple of specific events that are worthy of sharing in detail:

On June 24, eleven days after my first chemo treatment, our neighbors, Pete and Star Folco, had their annual "Guitar B-Q" party. It was a full day of music, sun, swimming in the pool, and laughter. I'm happy to recall it as a good day that even Lindsay and her new boyfriend, Lars, attended. Former neighbors, Jeff and Patty McCormack, also came and took part in the evening "jam" session around the campfire. Jeff had lived through lung cancer a few years prior and it was inspiring to see someone who had "come out on the other side" of this insidious disease. Maybe life would resume as normal.

On July 5, after my second treatment, Ken and I embarked on a five night, six day motorcycle trip to upper Michigan along with our friends, Kenny Preville, Patty and Jim Mitchell. Day one took us to Hale, Michigan, to visit Ken's sister, Nancy, and her family. We were treated to the local F.O.E. (Fraternal Order of Eagles) fish dinner, a massive fireworks display on the lake, and indoor sleeping accommodations for all. Day two we headed for the Mackinaw Bridge, the longest suspension bridge in the United States (between anchorages-meaning land mass). Two others are actually longer to meet the suspension span technicality (span between towers)—the Golden Gate Bridge in San Francisco and a new bay bridge in New York. Regardless of which one holds the title, the Mackinaw Bridge is thrilling and can be dangerous in high winds if a driver is not careful. The ride across the Bridge would take us to the "U-P" (that's what we Michiganians call the Upper Peninsula). Citizens living in the U.P. are "Yoopers" (due to the common Finnish accent for "UP-pers" and citizens living in the lower peninsula are "Trolls" (living under the bridge as in fairy tales) or "Apple Knockers" (deer hunters who bait white tail deer with piles of apples in the woods). It's all in fun.

After a tour of the Lumberjack Museum, lunch in Mackinaw City and picture-taking at the scenic view turn-out, we were at the bridge. We all agreed—no riding on the grate. For anyone unfamiliar with the spectacular Mackinaw Bridge, it is a five mile long, four lane bridge. One lane in each direction is paved like a regular road and one has a steel grate that allows you to see through to the water far below. We agreed a second time—no riding on the grate section. Being all "leathered" up in our riding gear, we had gotten our toll money out as we loaded up after lunch in Mackinaw City so as we approached the bridge, I clutched our money and anxiously looked ahead. Ya-hoo! We were all going to meet our goal of riding over the bridge on our new Harley Davidsons. We proceeded ahead. The cautionary words **HIGH WIND ADVISORY** flashed ominously on the overhead electronic message board! Patty and I smiled somewhat nervously back and forth. Oh well, we'd just seen other motorcycles come back from the other side, so we would be okay. Suddenly, bright orange highway marker cones appeared. What was going on? All along the paved lane of the bridge, orange cones were lined up. We had to ride the grate! Obviously, we made it; it wasn't that bad. I kind of equated this experience to the cancer. The water was scary below us and the wind fought us, but we had faith we could cross over it. And we did-on both trips (across the big Mackinaw Bridge and with the big C, cancer).

The trip proceeded and we set up camp by pitching our tents at a rustic campground (meaning no indoor plumbing, no running water or electricity). We hit the local grocery store and purchased essentials-water, snacks, juice, etc., made friends with the camp site host, gathered wood, and laughed around the fire for most of the night. But we did take a visit to the local casino and the adventure turned out fairly lucrative for three out of five of us (sorry Patty and Jimi). At least we all had breakfast the next morning "on the casino"!

Sleeping in the tents was great fun although it did occur to me (after dark) that there might be bears in this remote site; but we never, thankfully, had any join us in our camp. The next morning around 6:30 a.m., however, we awoke to tree limbs falling and loud squawking. While it felt, at first, like we were under attack, a quick run to the bathrooms identified the noise was just crows who flew away upon seeing us. Maybe we were in their morning breakfast spot.

After we packed up and had the aforementioned breakfast on our casino winnings, it was time to ride back across the big bridge and part ways. Ken and I were going to meet my parents and friends at Blissfest, an annual music festival near Cross Village, which is on the shore of Lake Michigan, and the rest of our 'gang' were going to take a scenic route back home to Lapeer.

Blissfest is a full weekend of folk and traditional music, communal camping, and camaraderie. We had gone several times before and it was always a great weekend. This trip raised one concern, however, due to the fact that I was ever diligent about exposing myself to any germs that might cause problems or delays with my treatment. All the information you read tells you to try not to delay treatment unless it is absolutely necessary because doing so could be detrimental to the eradication of the cancer. That concern was Port-o-Potties or Port-a-Johns, those charming plastic public outhouses seen at campsites and carnivals that don't rate high for sanitation in my estimation. So in our packing sessions, we had decided to erect my very own "Princess Potty Tent". It was a one person, stand up hunting blind in which we positioned a (special purchase) camping bucket complete with a toilet seat and lid—almost like home! It served its purpose and got us a few laughs, too.

The weekend was great. Old friends, Shelly McDonald, who lived a few miles away from the festival site, and Jeff McCormack, both cancer survivors, were able to join us for a couple days and help inspire me to recovery with their positive attitude and zest for life. Another old friend, the "Blissfest Apple Tree", the only scrap of shade on the viewing slope, made it safe for me to watch the stage for hours while sitting under its leafy branches. The sun shone some of the time, it was windy all of the time, and the rain fell although we were rewarded with the most brilliant double rainbow. We were like brilliantly colored flowers even in our temporary garden. Life, indeed, was proceeding with some normalcy.

***

MD:

Sounds of happiness, joyous laughter, easy-on-the-ears music and caring voices are therapeutic. They can affect your mood and emotional state in a positive way to promote healing. Your mind-set about your health and your willingness to work toward good health make a huge difference in beating cancer.

Dede made a conscious decision to stay in high spirits. This fact had great benefit for her and the whole family. I was so very proud of her. She had projects—re-organizing closets, redecorating activity in the house, and invited me to attend cancer fighter group meetings where we would meet many super nice people and would learn something new every where we went. She and her only child (and my only granddaughter-which makes her doubly precious to us) found a new level of mother and daughter relationship, spending more time together and letting their love for each other show in every action.

Much of the laughter found in the Garden of Being comes from friends and family. Dede received encouragement and an abundance of love and support from friends and family. Friends sent flowers, cards, emails and angel figurines. Friends who offered encouragement during Dede's treatment were angels of hope. Some of her closest pals, Patty Mitchell, Marti Hamilton, Elise McCullough, and Dorcas McIntosh, were extremely caring and also provided the perfect mix of humor, affection, and advice whenever the situation warranted.

Ken's Hammerberg family members provided love and support just as if she were one of them; actually, she was an "official" Hammerberg ever since her and Ken's wedding day on June 16, 2003. Her neighbors, Dave Oparka, Julie and Brian Jones, Sandy and Mike Ancona, Star and Pete Folco, and Sherry and Phil Adams were on "call" status if she would happen to need them. Love is powerful medicine.

One of her big preoccupations was writing proposals for a new career path which would include working in the healing arts, specifically in the oncology area to develop a resource program for ancillary, non-traditional cancer treatment that would encourage involvement in whole body regimens. She believed that it should not be so difficult for a cancer patient to have knowledge of and easy access to these resources. Dede had already formed a business concept for a personal services visit service for residents of assisted living facilities called Time Angels that she had not yet fully implemented due to her on-going treatment. There was potential to combine elements of that plan into her new mission. Dede is a force of nature and she was determined to not let cancer have the last word.

Blissfest is a music and folk art annual festival held in Bliss, Michigan, only 50 miles southwest of the Mackinaw Bridge. My husband and I had attended this remarkable event for three years. This year Dede and Ken had planned to join us and best friends of ours, David and Tawyna Stock (also Blissfest alumni), to set up our tents in a "compound" fashion. We named our campsite, The Magic Carpet Camp, decorating our common area in a slightly Arabian Nights tent style, although it was so extremely windy it looked rather like we were in a desert sandstorm with the side drapes wildly flapping and falling off. The gazebo type tent shelter actually blew over as a result of a fierce gust and we had to repair and redesign. It was a weekend of surprise, fun, and good company. It was a goal to race down to the stage area early in the day to make 'claim' for our tribe's blanket spot under the solitary apple tree, which provided just enough light shade. Amazingly, we were able to occupy this prized spot for the two day weekend. This apple tree beckons us each time we visit as an old friend might do. We like it and we believe it likes us, too.

A rare occurrence made that Saturday at Blissfest 2006 very memorable. It was windy, yet warm and raining lightly. We joined a crowd of about 300 other revelers under a big open tent to hear a terrific singer and musician, Harry Manx, who had the crowd under his spell. A bit of commotion happened when about a dozen people jumped out of the tent area, pointing and waving their arms excitedly toward the eastern sky. What we saw wasn't a UFO. It was even better- an awesome color prism rainbow stretching across a quarter width of the 360 degree sky with the rain still coming down softly. It made my heart stand still. For a brief spell, a double rainbow was seen. Some amorous couples danced in the rain under the rainbow, in soggy clothes but smiling. It was a state of bliss.

Laughter and music in the "Garden of Being" are the sounds of the phone ringing and then hearing a friendly voice on the line, hearing a favorite song running through your head, listening to the cat purr next to your ear, and sharing laughter and "I love you's" with special people.

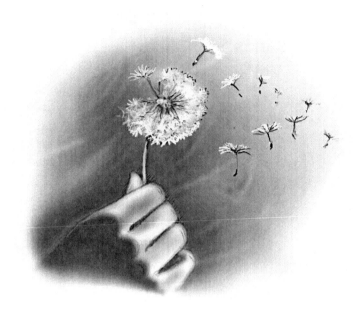

11

Garden of Wishes
and Dreams

MD:

I am so grateful that I am able to join and walk with my daughter on this 'unscheduled' garden tour of discovery and for her choosing the perfect title for this book, The Garden of Being.

At first, what I thought I heard Dede say was that she had suggested, Garden of "Be'an" for the title. What? I was thinking, well, "okey-dokey". It's funny, but it might work. We could compare human <u>beings</u> as representing all colors and land of origin <u>beans</u>—red beans, white beans, black beans, brown beans, yellow beans, green beans, navy beans, pinto beans, bean sprouts, and beige lentil beans! That seemed to fit into the garden grown theme nicely. We could refer to the human be'an condition as- fresh, steamed, mushy, refried, dried, baked, frozen, 'lie'-ma beans, clinging vine, 'kid'-ney beans, string beans, bush or peanut (peanuts are not a true "nut", but from the bean family) and "porky" beans! I have met people who would fit all those descriptions. But, luckily, her original idea, although I did not hear correctly it at first, was <u>much</u> better. I need to get my hearing checked.

I have always felt that part of our "immortality" is when we pass tiny bits of our own love and spirit between those we love or to those we connect with as friends. The recipients, in turn, pass on these tiny bits of love as good deeds, like dandelion seed "parachutes" floating in the air, until they find a fertile place to take root and perform their miraculous cycle all over again in exponential fashion. What we do, or do not do, today has impact on humans, the environment, and our gardens for as far as we can see into the future.

Gardens are not just to grow flowers and vegetables; gardens are to grow people's wishes and dreams and to help people grow their appreciation of all living organisms, especially themselves.

Think of your body and your life as a garden. If you do not plan and tend to your garden of being, it will turn to a weed patch, full of useless and harmful things. What gardens have in common with us is that they are all about life and living.

The title of this book, The Garden of Being, is symbolic of the human condition and for the wellspring of belief in the personal power we have in our own healing and the fact that we are indeed surrounded by a garden of life.

Our planet earth is a garden and all that applies to making a garden healthy and productive is the same for our earth. God, whoever and wherever you are, please show us in a way that leaves no doubt, how to take care of our precious gardens.

In my Garden of Wishes and Dreams, some things in life would be different. For instance, I am highly skeptical of the pharmaceutical industry at large. The name of this game, as with most mega-corporations, is profit over social conscience. Profit itself, is not evil, but profit at expense of providing the public with safe, effective and affordable medicine is evil. The system of "inventing" new miracle drugs that are usually (and conveniently) fast-track approved by Federal Drug Administration for sale to the public, marketed and glamorized by million dollar TV and print advertising is a sick system. Some of the major fiascos like Vioxx® had not been given adequate trial and resulted in many deaths. Other suspected killer drugs, Bextra® and Celebrex® remain on the market as of this date, although with "Black Box Warnings" on retail packaging about possible adverse reactions. My husband had close calls with the use of Lipitor® and Aldara® which resulted in doctor and emergency room visits. Don't count on the FDA to monitor the safety of new drugs. The FDA is lobbied intensely by "Big Pharma" to get new potential money making drugs to market quickly. The consumer (that's us) needs to be constantly vigilant.

So many of our physical ills could be prevented and likely cured with good nutrition and eating habits. We are a society of pill addicts, always looking for a "magic pill" to compensate for our own personal neglect and abuse.

The tragedy is that we, the consumers, buy into the hype and hope of these new and fashionable drugs to cure whatever ails us. Is it "brainwashing" or our own ignorance? Getting back to basics to help our body cure itself as much as possible is a sensible goal. Nature intended nutrients in plants and animals to provide humans with nutrition needed to function. The challenge today is to find food sources that are untainted by harmful preservatives, toxins and bacteria. Don't count on the United States Department of Agriculture to do it. The USDA is intensely lobbied by mega food producers to keep oversight to a minimum. Safety in food packaging and production is not as carefully monitored as it should be. That is why contaminated food gets into the network and ends up poisoning people.

The FDA and USDA, as many government institutions, are highly influenced by corporate lobby groups; and for the most part, are not working for the public benefit, but for personal benefit. I wish it was not true and ask myself, "What can I do?" I am trying to figure that one out. I think it can start with writing letters. As voting citizens, we can be the strongest lobby group in the country.

We, as individuals, are responsible for what we eat and drink (and smoke). As for the air we breathe, that may be another matter. But it is true that bad habits and behaviors can hurt our physical health and may "invite" cancer to take root in our bodies. Healthy food and habits can help us to heal and avoid disease. I have learned a lot about eating healthier recently. Having grown up on saturated fat-based margarine, white bread, sugar-coated cereal and cookies, it's a "wonder" to me I survived all the "wonder" bread I ate that was missing whole grains and fiber!

My cynicism (almost) makes me feel guilty about thinking that major non-profit mega-size foundations/organizations who are in the business of finding a cure for cancer, diabetes, and other diseases aren't really trying hard enough. Is money raised going to research? These organizations raise thousands and thousands of dollars, yet we have not heard of their efforts resulting in any major discoveries to eradicate these diseases. It makes me wonder—why? It seems these mega-money raising institutions are more geared to self-sustaining bureaucratic existence than in finding "cures".

As individuals we must take blame for some of the problems mentioned about food and drug safety. We can make a difference (or not) in the following ways:

- We can choose to buy—or not to buy (one dollar = one vote)
- We can choose to vote—or not to vote
- We can choose to learn—or not to learn
- We can choose to think—or not to think
- We can write our representatives in government on important issues—or not

The "choose to" options might save us from further disaster. The "or not" choice will not give us much chance to see any positive changes.

Label the following as of "**Utmost Importance**": The ruling by United States Patent Office upon a court decision that genomes (DNA codes for specific gene activity) can be patented and be the intellectual property of someone is horrendous (and I believe not to be legally enforceable). Genes and DNA are facts of life and have not been "invented", only revealed. It is like giving someone an exclusive patent on the chemical composition for air or water. This ruling should be overturned in the interest of humanity. If scientists are able to reveal the gene that causes cancer and one entity has exclusive patent rights and sets the price at a $1,000,000.00, what next? It is not going to help many cancer patients, only millionaires.

Our Garden of Wishes and Dreams can be planted, tended, and encouraged to grow into a bountiful and healthy garden with care and caution. Let us try.

Toward the 'finish-up' phase of this book collaboration, I remembered a sweet story from my childhood that I had not thought about for over fifty years. I told Dede I wanted to read it again; and maybe she would like to read it, too. The book is The Secret Garden by Frances Hodgson Burnett, first published in 1911. Dede went to the Lapeer library that same day. Lo and behold, a copy was sitting there, waiting for us to check it out!

The story line is magical. It is about attitude 'adjustment' and life transformation from negative to positive. It relates to a person's health and personality 'blooming' with encouragement just like the sun and rain nourish the garden. A young girl, Mary, is orphaned and sent to live with an uncle in England. She has a sour disposition and finds life joyless. Through the positive influences of the manor's staff and her discovery of a hidden "secret garden" on the grounds, her life takes an entire new and positive direction. In the process, she helps her cousin, the invalid son of her uncle, attain a miraculous recovery. Bringing the hidden garden back to life and renewed beauty is a central theme of the story. The moral of the story is that there is indeed "magic" in life and how important it is to give things room and a little bit of help to grow.

***

DD:

I, too, am so grateful that I was able to have my mother walk beside me on this garden tour of discovery of what is truly important in life.

We, as humans, are interdependent upon each other just like the flowers or plants in your garden. Cultivate relationships with the ones that are the most important for your own ecological 'balance'. Weed out the picker weeds and 'crab' grass that saps your energy and help nurture those that support you. And, most of all, love and care for each other. When you do, your garden, too, will be full yet have enough room to grow your wishes and dreams.

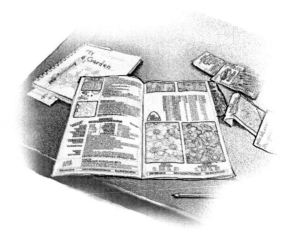

Planning for
Next Year's Garden

Happiness (Old Chinese Proverb)
If you want to be happy for an hour, roast a pig.
If you want to be happy for a year, marry.
If you want to be happy for a lifetime, plant a garden.

MD:

A fun part of gardening is planning how you will do it better next year! Seed and garden supply catalogs appear in our mailbox as early as December, even before Christmas! I swear they take pictures of wax fruit and vegetables because I've never been able to grow anything that looks quite as perfect as shown in the catalog photos, but that does not mean I will stop trying. A garden, large or small, can always be visualized as more productive, more colorful and more aesthetically arranged—next year. Mother Nature seems to be happy to give us another chance to get it right. Life is like that, too. There is always room for improvement.

Thinking about next summer's garden (even if it will be a tomato plant or two sitting in pots on the deck) during the frigid, snowy Michigan winter helps to keep my 'gardening spirit' pacified. I plan to rethink our garden spaces and how to make them appealing during the snow months—maybe with red bark shrubs for color contrast or brightly colored bird feeders (which may attract brightly colored feathered friends). Learning to appreciate the beauty of nature within the changing seasons is perhaps like learning to appreciate our physical life's "seasons" of age and health. People, like plants and trees, need seasons of rest and cycles of low and high productivity. I recall reading about an ancient myth of the "Green Man" who is symbolized as a human face growing within a crown head of green plants and foliage. The image, sculptured and painted, appears frequently in Grecian and Roman architecture. Ancient people felt that man and nature were closely related. So do I. I believe nature is us and we are nature.

"Victory" gardens were encouraged by the U. S. government in the mid-1940's following WWII. Many families that had garden space did so both out of patriotism, but more out of necessity as food was expensive and in short supply for the middle and lower class population. I remember my grandmother's garden in Flint, Michigan's north end when I was nine years old in 1949. It was about 20 by 30 feet in size. A neighbor would plow it initially one time. From then on it was entirely hand tilled and tended. The soil was poor, mostly clay, but grandma managed to grow beans, tomatoes, beets, onions, and cucumbers which she "put up"(canned) in glass mason jars for the winter. I think the word "victory" meant having enough food to stay alive during the hard times. Our personal "Garden of Being", our mind-body-spirit entity, can be our own "victory" as expressed through our life and legacy.

Cherish your second chances and new opportunities.

***

DD:

We had received our miracle, **remission**! The scans were clear. Yes, there were still treatments to go through, but life was sweet. It's funny how my seasons had been turned upside down this year. Here it was November and this day was the sunniest, warmest day of the year.

Planning not only for 'the' future but for 'a' future is priceless. It is said that there is a time for everything. I believe this to be true, but I have to say that my favorite season is 'planning', the time of the season when anything is possible. You may not see it, but the sun is shining during 'planning season'. The clouds are only temporarily in the way.

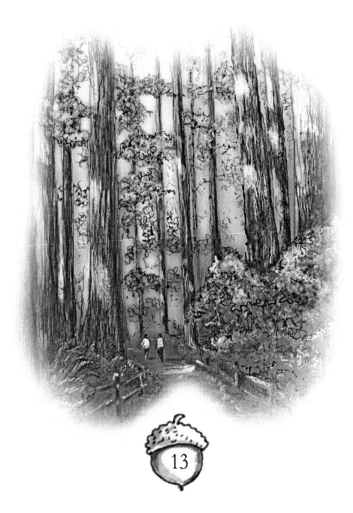

13

Celebration Garden

DD:

Our trip to San Francisco was exactly what I needed in cold, cold February 2007. Even a slight delay in our original departure flight due to a winter storm couldn't put a damper on the trip. The weather was atypical San Francisco weather. I didn't miss it really, but where was the fog and drizzle I had been warned about? As always (see chapter 7), I felt the ol' Dede luck paving the way for a delightful trip.

Of all the exciting, wonderful things we did, the best for me was sharing time with Dorcas. We had become spiritual friends many years prior and she was definitely one of the people I needed to celebrate my victory with. Having my mother to be a part of the celebration made the whole circle complete. And I was now able to see why Dorcas was so drawn to this area. She fit in, this Michigan sweet cherry tree, with the potted jade plants and multitude of flowering trees of San Francisco perfectly. And, we were able, for a short time, to visit and admire the beauty of her new garden. We were lucky enough to get to meet her sons, Ben, Bruno and Tim, for the first time, too. Dorcas' sons reflect her spirit of love and generosity. Watching the interaction and love between Dorcas and her sons reminded me that as a gardener "mom", she must feel so proud of having 'grown' such wonderful human "be'ans". (Okay, mom, we get to use the 'be'an' joke again).

***

MD:

At the conclusion of Dede's six-month chemotherapy, we decided to do something big for us to celebrate. We chose to visit San Francisco in February 2007. Dede's close friend,

Dorcas McIntosh, recently moved there and graciously offered her apartment's extra bedroom for us to use. She could call her apartment the <u>Two</u> Bee's (B & B for Bed & Breakfast) as she has frequent house guests like us two country bumpkins wanting to visit the most famous California city by the bay!

We had a fantastic time. The weather was sunny and dry every day! Dede boasted that we took along our 'good weather insurance policy' (umbrellas and rain ponchos—which were unused). We saw the major sights—the Golden Gate Bridge, the elegant downtown district, took a trolley ride, saw a musical revue, "Beach Blanket Babylon", visited Fisherman's Wharf, ate like thieves and even accompanied Dorcas to work for a day at her son's business, Three Bees Nursery on Clement Street in the Richmond District. We tried to be useful in between "oohing" and "ahhhing" at the beautiful plants and flowers. As I observed visitors to the nursery meander around the arrangements, it was as if we humans, of all ethnic backgrounds, have a need to 'commune' with nature. It is as if the plants are giving off an 'energy' that enters our body and mind and somehow re-energizes us.

One day Dorcas drove us to Muir Woods just north of Sausalito. It was an extraordinary day! Muir Woods, named in honor of naturalist John Muir, contains the world's most famous redwoods—some more than 1,000 years old. It was awe inspiring. When we first entered the park, it was like stepping into a garden of giants. The majestic redwoods seemed to touch the clouds. The scene took my breath away. Dorcas pointed out an amazing habit of the redwoods. There were many clusters of trees in circular formations that are formed as a result of when a solitary tree is dying (lightning strike or diseased), the support roots send up 'soldier saplings' to encircle the 'fallen' tree and grow anew. This phenomenon seemed to represent the 'circle of life' for the magnificent and ageless trees. In human terms, the circle growth pattern of the redwoods made me think of human 'roots' and the life perpetuating strength of friends and family and our progeny who will take their space on this earth when the life force of our bodies is depleted. As I have felt the stimulating energy force from a display of small live plants, the energy force from the giant redwoods is invigorating to the mind and body on a magnificent scale.

We stopped at the gift shop in the park and happened on an oversize postcard bearing a poem that seemed perfectly attuned to what we had just "felt" the giant redwood trees saying to us as we marveled at their strength and beauty. The author, Ilan Shamir, kindly has given permission for us to share it with our readers (see copyright information that follows poem).

Advice From a Tree®
Dear Friend,
Stand Tall and Proud
Sink your Roots deeply into the Earth
Reflect the light of your own true nature
Think long term
Go out on a limb
Remember your place among all living beings
For each yields its own abundance
The Energy and Birth of Spring
The Growth and Contentment of Summer
The Wisdom to let go like leaves in the Fall
The Rest and Quiet Renewal of Winter
Feel the wind and the sun
And delight in their presence
Look up at the moon that shines down upon you
And the mystery of the stars at night
Seek nourishment from the good things in life
Simple pleasures
Earth, Fresh Air, Light
Be Content with your natural beauty
Drink plenty of Water
Let your limbs sway and dance in the breezes
Be flexible
Remember your Roots!
Enjoy the View!

Ilan Shamir

As we three women walked the winding path beside the crystal clear, gurgling river stream, we talked about how listening to sounds of flowing water and gazing at the dancing flames of a campfire can focus our mind to the basic life forces in nature—water, fire, earth and wind. It was a magical day. How grand is our Garden.

We should cultivate our Garden of Being to be a "celebration" garden of wonderful memories.

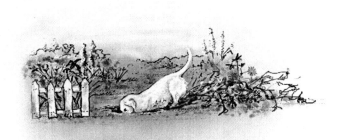

14

Garden Tips

Garden Tips

- Plant seeds of kindness everywhere you go; the seeds will take root and flower. This will become your legacy.

- Play in the dirt every chance you get; keep your inner child at play.

- Take time to stop and smell the roses, lavender, peppermint, rosemary, etc.

- Don't let weeds in your garden ruin your day; weeds are like out-of-control children who scream incessantly for attention. Ignoring them isn't always the best action. Acknowledge them and deal with them firmly.—Dolly Arksey

Following sayings are from internet inspirational message sites. Quote source anonymous or unknown unless shown:

- He who would have nothing to do with thorns must never attempt to gather flowers.

- What sunshine is to flowers, smiles are to humanity. Go often to the house of your friend, for weeds choke up the unused path.

- The foolish man seeks happiness in the distance; the wise man grows it under his feet. Happiness is in our own backyard.

- A peck of common sense is worth a bushel of learning.

- Today's profits are yesterday's goodwill ripened.

- Gardening, like old age, isn't for sissies.

- If you won't plow in the cold, you won't eat at the harvest (Proverbs 20:4)

- The harvest I reap is measured by the attitudes I cultivate—Iyanla Van Zant

- Hug a tree; everybody needs a hug now and then.

- You can bury a lot of troubles digging in the dirt.

- Gardening requires lots of water-most of it in the form of perspiration.- Lois Erickson

- A garden is the best alternate therapy.—Germaine Greer

- The family that rakes together, aches together.

- Plant a seed of friendship; reap a bouquet of happiness.—Lois L. Kaufman

- Never go to a doctor whose office plants have died.— Sir Francis Bacon

- Leave room in your garden for angels to dance.

- Gardening: Just another day at the plant!—Elizabeth Lawrence

- Give your weeds an inch and they'll take your yard.—Edgar A. Guest

- In order to live off a garden, you practically have to live in it.—Frank McKinney Hubbard

- Bloom where you are planted. J. C. Raulston

- Love this Earth as if you won't be here tomorrow; show reverence for your Garden as if you will be here forever.—Scottish Proverb

- The gardening bug can bite at any moment.—Karel Capek

- Our bodies are our gardens . . our wills are our gardeners.—William Shakespeare.

- Gardening adds years to your life and life to your years.

- The most important garden tool is one you won't find at the hardware store, but is an absolute necessity-a sense of humor.

- Location, location, location—is also true for plants—Michael P. Garofalo

- Where flowers bloom, there is hope.—Lady Bird Johnson

***

Garden Jokes:

- Q: How do you fix a broken tomato?
  A: With tomato paste!

- "Don't bend over in the garden, Granny. You know them tater's got eyes!"

- Flowers grow by inches, but are destroyed by feet.

- First law of holes: If you are in one, stop digging.—Denis Healy

- Gardeners learn by trowel and error.—Unknown

- If you are a gardener, you can put "Plant Manager" on your resume.—Unknown

- Old gardeners never die, they just run out of thyme.—Unknown

- Q: What do you call it when worms take over the world?
  A: Global worming

- Q. Where do vegetables go to have a few drinks?
  A: The Salad Bar

- Q: What are the four seasons?
  A: Salt, pepper, mustard, vinegar

- Q: What do you get if you divide the circumference of a pumpkin by its diameter?
  A: Pumpkin pi

- Q: What can you make from baked beans and onions?
  A: Tear gas

- Q: Why do potatoes make good detectives?
  A: Because they keep their eyes peeled

- Q: What kind of socks does a gardener wear?
  A: Garden hose

***

Words of Advice From the Garden:

Life is like a garden. You reap just what you sow. All you tend with loving care will multiply and grow. So plant some "peas" called pleasantness, praise and patience, too. Those qualities just sparkle like grass wet with morning dew. "Lettuce" not be so competitive with people that we meet. Your fellow man is not someone you need to "squash" or "beet". "Turnip" that joy, share a hug, put on a sunny grin, for what sprouts in life's great garden are the seeds that you put in!—Author Unknown (but it may have been spoken by a real "human be'an")

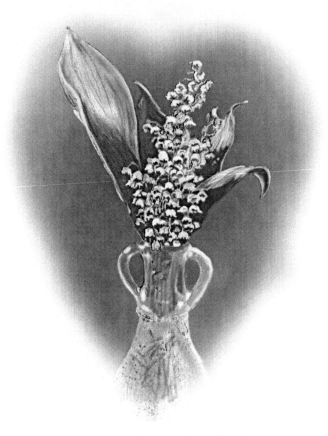

Message from the Authors

MD:

"Look deep into nature, and then you will understand everything better"-Albert Einstein.

My daughter's message that concludes this story speaks for us both. On a personal note, I want her to know that she continues to help me aspire to be worthy of the title of motherhood and that she fills my heart with love and pride We are learning many things together, the most important is that life can be so fragile, but love makes us strong.

This has been almost a full year of the experience we call "life" and has profoundly changed my perception of the world around me. It seems that I think "deeper" and "feel" more intensely. I wish to be more of an 'activist' in those issues that affect the whole of the earth and all human beings. I wish to be free- "Free" of mind to question everything and criticize everything in a productive way. I wish not to be "told" what to think. An open mind is the solution, I believe, to many problems. It may be due to my having entered further into the phase of my life as a senior citizen and knowing that likely the useful years remaining for me number less than my total count of fingers and toes. That reality, coupled with the extraordinary experience of the past year that involved my daughter's cancer battle, is responsible for the new direction in my thinking. It seems a shame that the freedom to have an 'open mind' is usually only granted to the very young or the very old without too much harassment or criticism.

***

DD:

> *"Every blade of grass has its angel that bends over it*
> *and whispers, "Grow, grow"*
> *-The Talmud*

Thank you for letting us share our journey with you. It is not a journey anyone would ask to go on and it is one I hope you never have to take. But if you do, take comfort in knowing that you have control over at least one part of your recovery— your attitude. It can make or break you.

- Your soil can become polluted by poor nutrition but it can become rich once again with the proper diet and nutrition.

- Your leaves can become infected with blight or other leaf rot but they can become lush and green again with the right treatments for your disease.

- Your stalk can wilt from lack of water but by hydrating yourself with clean, clear water you can become strong and hardy again.

- Your blooms can become faded and tough from too much sun but with the help of shade from your friends and loved ones you can blossom and be bright once more.

I've learned a lot on this journey. Cancer is not, always, the thief of life we've come to know it as. Cancer is a chronic disease, just like diabetes. It can, in many cases, be something we live <u>with</u> instead of die <u>from</u>. None of us, patient or doctor, are God. And none of us know when the privilege of life is going to be taken from us. We are lucky when we realize this and live our lives to the fullest, letting love and laughter be the predominant tone of our life. As the song says, 'Go skydiving, rocky mountain climbing', whatever your heart yearns for, do. None of us are guaranteed tomorrow; let us learn to live, not with the fear, but the promise.

Life can be harsh, just like a long, cold Alaskan winter. It can also be warm and comforting, like the bright California sun. Wherever you are planted, learn to live with the elements, not against them. May your garden bloom with perpetual bliss.

A personal discovery I've made when I am reading a good book is that "music can be found in the written word". I hope you have 'heard' some music to your liking while reading this book.

With love and care always—

Dede Hammerberg

ABOUT THE AUTHORS

Denise (Dede) Hammerberg

Denise lives in Lapeer, Michigan, and is married to Kenneth Hammerberg. She has one daughter, Lindsay Anne Martin. Her work history includes positions as collections agent and several years of managerial assignments in the automotive supplies industry. Her favorite pastimes are crafting, gardening, and trips with her husband Ken on their Harley Davidson motorcycle. After her diagnosis of stage IV breast cancer in 2006, writing became therapy as well as a new creative outlet. Her journey through chemotherapy led to a "miracle" of full cancer remission in early 2007. She is inspired to help other cancer patients with encouragement and example. The book, The Garden of Being, is the first 'fruit' from her "Inspiration Tree". A children's book, also with a garden theme, will soon be in publication.

Dorla (Dolly) Arksey

Dolly grew up in Flint, Michigan, but has lived in Lapeer, Michigan, since 1964. She is married to Richard Arksey and has two children, Denise and Dennis, and two grandchildren, Lindsay and Michael. Her work history includes positions as secretary, real estate agent/broker, and Irish Pub owner/manager. Writing books has been 'teasing' her mind for a long time. She has completed two manuscripts and co-authored "The Garden of Being" with her daughter, Denise. She has three other book projects in process and works on these according to the prevailing "mood" of the day.

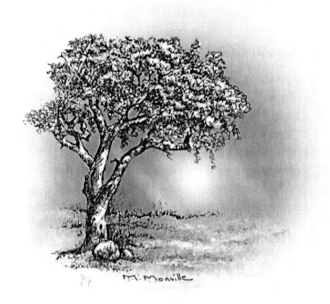

MIKE MONVILLE
Artist/Illustrator

Mike Monville is a self-taught artist and credits a curious mind and the public library system throughout the State of Michigan for his education in the visual arts. He works in several media, including pencil, ink, watercolor, pastel and acrylic paint as well as clay and metal sculpture. His works are held in many private and public collections in the United Sates and abroad.

Mike teaches drawing classes based on the 'Drawing on the Right Side of the Brain' techniques pioneered by Dr. Betty Edwards of California State University at Long Beach. He also teaches pen and ink drawing and watercolor painting—at his "Three Waters Studio" and at the Gallery 194/Lapeer Center for the Arts in the city of Lapeer, Michigan.

The theme of Mike's work is inspired by nature—animals, birds, trees, plant life, and landscapes. His home and studio are surrounded by nature's abundance which serves as the source for many of his paintings and drawings. Mike and his wife, Donna, a crafts artist specializing in basket weaving, beeswax candles, "Bee Skeps" and pottery, reside in rural Lapeer County, Michigan, where they operate the Three Waters Studio. Their homestead and nature haven is aptly named Critter Creek.

RECOMMENDED READING

How to Fight Cancer and Win   William L. Fischer
A comprehensive and encouraging book on alternative
and ancillary cancer treatments and cancer prevention
with strong focus on nutrition and naturopathy.

There's No Place Like Hope   Vickie Gerard
A personal and inspiration 'guide book' written by a
courageous and determined woman who became an
inspiration to thousands of cancer patients.

The Secret Garden   Francis Burgett Hodgson
A classic around since early 1900's geared to youth,
but story and lessons applicable to all ages. It is a
charming and timeless story of the healing power
of positive attitude and love of nature. It has been
adapted as a stage play.

Silent Spring   Rachel Carson
Celebrated award winning expose on effects of
chemical contamination of our environment (first
published 1962). Written by a scientist and renown
conservationist, it should be required reading by all
public officials, especially United State Department
of Agriculture; Department of Natural Resources;
college students taking Biology and Chemistry; and,
basically, everyone able to read.

Bambi   Felix Salten

This novel, originally published in 1929 and translated from its original German edition, is the story of the life of a young deer from his birth to the death of his father and simultaneous birth of his own offspring. Eloquently written, the descriptions of each animal show their unique personalities and brings them alive to the reader. It shows throughout how connected all life forms are to nature and each other. Appropriate for ages seven to seventy and beyond.

Fighting Cancer and   Annette & Richard Bloch
Guide for Cancer Supporters

Informative, easy to read, step-by-step guides to help cancer patients and caregivers fight cancer. Both were written by cancer survivor, Richard Bloch, and his wife after he successfully beat lung cancer in 1980 and are available without charge by calling 1-(800) 433-0464 or visiting the website www.blochcancer. org.

Beating Cancer with Nutrition   Patrick Quillin,
PhD, RD, CNS, with Noreen Quillin

A terrific technical book which outlines the importance of good nutrition in the fight against cancer. Of particular interest are the <u>Rating Your Foods</u> chart found on the last page and a CD narrated by the authors.

A Mindful Life   Vivekanand Palavali, M.D.

A neurosurgeon reflects on how he overcame an obsession with dying as a young man and learned to express a beautiful humanistic wisdom about life. Stories of real life medical dramas with which the doctor was involved convey the message of being mindful of cherishing all that life offers us in the present.

Cancer-Step Outside the Box   Ty M. Bollinger

The author is not a medical doctor, but has done extensive research as to available alternate cancer treatments. He was motivated to research this subject in memory of his father and mother who both died of cancer, under similar diagnoses and a short interval apart. His book is critical of the major players in the medical, pharmaceutical, and research/support alliances that support only 'traditional' remedies prescribed by the medical profession for cancer treatment. His book is highly thought provoking, promoting the idea that cancer patients need to know all their choices. He is outspoken about the dismal survival statistics of current cancer treatments and the need for innovations and a new direction in fighting cancer.

Made in the USA